Food Fight!

Amanda,
Wishing you
peace & joy
with food.
Dawn

Food Fight!

Ending the Struggle Once and for All

Dawn MacLaughlin, PhD

Food Fight! Ending the Struggle Once and for All
Copyright © 2017 by Dawn MacLaughlin, PhD

ISBN: 197917671X
ISBN 13: 9781979176712

Note: The information in this book is true and complete to the best of our knowledge. The book is intended only as an informative guide for those wishing to know more about changing their relationship with food. In no way is this book intended to replace, countermand, or conflict with advice given to you by your licensed physician, dietician, or nutritionist. The ultimate decision concerning your care should be made by you in consultation with your doctor. Information in this book is general and is offered with no guarantees on the part of the author or the publisher. The author and publisher disclaim all liability in connection with the use of this book.

To everyone who has struggled with food,
who has lived that constant, draining battle.
It's time to stop fighting.
I know you have much better things to do.

To my friends and family and coaches and colleagues
who have supported me as I've navigated my own
food fight—I thank you.

To my mother—I miss you every day.

To my husband—you are my rock.

Contents

One

My Food Fight

Not again…

Ugh.

I'm sitting in my car in a parking lot. There's no one parked near me. Apparently, I parked away from the crowd.

My fingers feel sticky. I look down to see crumbs all over me. In the passenger seat is an empty plastic tray that just moments ago held some number of cupcakes. I assume there were four because I count four empty cupcake wrappers in the tray. And I see remnants of frosting. It looks like I used a finger to get at the frosting that had come into contact with the tray. I can see a distinct swirl in the frosting remnant.

What the hell is wrong with me? How could I let this happen again?

I mean, I had told myself the minute I got up this morning that today would be different. Today would be the day I would break the cycle. I'd just go to work, do my job—and do it well—and then come home, feeling proud of myself because I didn't do it again. I'd cook dinner and sit down and eat it with my husband. I'd bring a healthy appetite to the table, and I'd enjoy the food. We'd talk about our days and then maybe watch some TV, relax, and read before retiring.

I'd even visualized my drive home—staying in the left lane, not the right, to help keep me from making that turn toward the cupcake store.

Yet here I am. Again.

As I realize that I have once again failed to break the cycle, that I have once again been unable to stop myself from doing this, the frustration and shame wash over me. I feel a sense of hopelessness. I am afraid that I will be forever stuck in this pattern.

"OK, pull yourself together," I say to myself. "Nothing you can do about the past. What's done is done. Gotta move on. Gotta get home and cook dinner and pretend like nothing is wrong."

And so I dust off the crumbs, clean up the frosting, and drive home, stopping somewhere along the way to throw out this trash. I manage to put forward a face of normalcy, even manage to eat dinner despite feeling full and bloated. But all I really want to do is crawl into bed and cry.

After all, tomorrow is another day. Another battle.

That used to be a typical day for me. Although I was never officially diagnosed, I know I was suffering from binge-eating disorder (BED). These binges would happen three or four—or more—times a week, week after week: cupcakes, cookies, cake, or peanut butter out of the jar. That last one was the one that finally got me caught—or rather, that got me to confess about my challenge to my husband. I mean, you can only go so long without a good explanation as to why the peanut butter keeps disappearing from the house. Especially when you two are the only people living there.

At the time, I was working for Weight Watchers as a meeting leader. I would go to work and lead meetings where I would counsel people—mostly women—on how to work the Weight Watchers system so they could eat less, move more, and lose weight. And then afterward I would binge. Whether it was driving to a cupcake store or a grocery store, I would consume a couple thousand calories of sugar and fat in a sitting, usually right there in my car. As you will see, my role as a Weight Watchers leader and the binge eating were not unrelated.

I don't know if you've ever experienced binge eating. For those who have not, it's hard to understand. Advising someone "Just don't do that" doesn't work. For me, binge eating was an out-of-body experience. During a binge, it felt like my body was taken over by some other controlling force. I could observe what was happening, as if from the sidelines, but I was helpless to interfere. And what was happening was that my body was rapidly and voraciously consuming food. There was no enjoyment. There was no pleasure. There was just a strong need to fill up. Sometimes my body would eat so rapidly that I would almost choke.

I learned that the binge mind is quite crafty. I used to refer to my binge persona as my FAD, or food addict demon. I hated that aspect of me. I wanted to exorcise it. It felt like a demonic spirit was exerting control—sometimes subtly, sometimes all out. And it got very creative in allowing me to binge without getting caught. I remember hearing it tell me things like "If you get four cupcakes, it will look like you're buying for the family, not yourself. Yep, four's a good number," or "You want to get a variety of options from the bakery to make it look like you're buying for a group." It had me drive to a different parking lot from where I bought the food so I could consume it without being seen. It had me hide food in my office. Hide wrappers in the trash. Even try to make the peanut butter jar look like there was still a lot left by swirling it around and up the middle!

So how did my binge eating develop? And what did I do to put it behind me? (Yes, I have put it behind me.)

To understand what contributed to my binge eating, we have to first visit my childhood.

I grew up in an environment of stress and fear and scarcity. My father was an angry alcoholic, and I was very much afraid of him. I remember lying in bed at night listening to him yelling, afraid of what I might wake up to the next day. Imagine being afraid to go to sleep because you aren't sure what you might wake up to!

Thankfully, my parents divorced when I was about six years old. Soon afterward, my father left the state to avoid paying child support. My mother worked several jobs to make ends meet. As the only girl of three children (I was the middle child), as soon as I was old enough, it fell upon me to help take care of the house. I learned to cook and clean and take care of my little brother. And I also learned to use food to manage the emotions I was feeling at that age: stress, resentment, anger, and others.

While I grew up heavier than the other kids my age (and yes, I was bullied about it, although we didn't call it bullying back then), I never experienced binge eating like I did as an adult. I went on to college (bachelor's from MIT, PhD from Boston University), got married (thirty years and counting!), and held some well-paying jobs in academia and the software industry. My husband and I both earned decent salaries, which allowed us to fairly quickly pay off student loans and purchase a home. We were your typical middle-class family. I enjoyed food. I loved to cook and dine out. I slowly and steadily gained weight, simply because I was eating too much for what my body needed. But I was happy.

And then began the pressure to diet. My doctor wanted me to lose weight. I had been experiencing some knee pain. I was told my blood pressure and cholesterol were too high and that losing weight was going to fix all that. So she prescribed Fen-Phen (a weight-loss drug that was later taken off the market). Well, I didn't lose weight, but I did develop a heart murmur. So next it was off to the nutritionist to begin counting calories. Then exchanges. I would lose some weight, but I couldn't sustain the regimen, and I'd gain it back.

I began to feel the frustration of dieting. Nothing I did was working! And it was so hard! I felt like I was a failure. My doctor told me these things would help me lose weight, but they didn't. Of course, I would later learn that it wasn't that I had failed; it was that the diets had failed me.

So I took a dieting hiatus for a while. I went back to being my normal, healthy, happy self.

And then came the "precipitating event."

People love to talk about precipitating events whenever transformation is involved. They'll ask, "What was the precipitating event that made you turn things around?" As if one moment is the spark of big change. I find the phrase "turn things around" to be interesting. It implies I was headed in a wrong direction. I don't see it that way at all. I was on my path, my journey, the one my soul was choosing to pursue. What others view as precipitating events, I prefer to view as encounters that influence the way I walk my path. With that in mind, here's a significant encounter that altered my path.

We moved from Massachusetts to Florida in December 2005. In April 2006, I got a phone call from my mother (who lived about ninety minutes away). She told me she had been diagnosed with stage IV ovarian cancer. It was one of those phone calls where you just can't quite process what is being said. Her doctors had a treatment program planned for her, and they believed she would live at least another year, perhaps longer. I'm sure there was more conversation, but I just don't remember.

When I hung up the phone, I felt like my world fell out from underneath me. I collapsed on the floor, curled into a ball, and began sobbing. I felt like I was caught in a tornado. Thoughts were swirling around in my head, but I wasn't able to hold on to any of them. It wasn't fair. She was only sixty-three. She'd always seemed healthy. She was just starting to build a comfortable life for herself after working so hard for so long. I was planning to spend time with her. We were going to do all kinds of fun things together. How could this happen? Why hadn't they figured this out sooner?

And then her treatment began. The multiple rounds of chemo interspersed with spinal injections and radiation treatments. Watching as she lost all her hair (eyebrows, eyelashes, everything) and fought through nausea and weakness, I felt helpless. On her good days, we'd act like everything was OK. Then on her bad days, the best I could do was to support her in whatever way I could. And man, she was such a trooper. I watched her be incredibly strong and positive. She was convinced she would beat it (or at least that's what she told us). Her courage and determination were inspirational.

Watching her fight so hard for her health, I began to realize how precious health was—and how precious life was. Recalling my own doctor's words—and the memes that society teaches us—I became convinced that being in a large body was very unhealthy and that I needed to do something about it right away. (It should be noted that my mother was never overweight, and aside from high blood pressure, I was medically healthy and fit.) And so, in January 2007, I joined Weight Watchers.

And you know what? I was actually able to stick with it. I counted my points. I made changes. I deprived myself. I attended my meetings regularly. And I lost weight. "The program works if you work the program." That was the mantra that was instilled in me. My success—every weigh-in that showed a loss—was celebrated. Again and again. That celebration, it's like a drug. You feel good. You get those feel good hormones circulating through you, and you want more. I rode that "success high" all the way to a "healthy" weight. I felt I was finally being acknowledged, appreciated, and valued. I was praised in the meeting room and outside by friends and family. My mom was very happy for me (although she often told me I was losing too much weight). I had never received so much praise and recognition. Not when I graduated from MIT. Not when I got my PhD. Only when I became skinny.

Now most people would see my journey with Weight Watchers as a tremendous success. I successfully lost weight! But the trick is what happens after. I have to tell you, I was terrified of regaining, so I kept attending meetings. I became obsessed with food. I couldn't just go out to eat, but I had to prepare and analyze and work to make sure I made a good choice. I avoided the "bad" foods as much as I could. I maintained my weight loss for a year. I felt great. I was still riding the success high. I was still being recognized for my great achievement on a regular basis. I wanted others to experience what I was feeling. I made the decision to join Weight Watchers as an employee so I could help others achieve the same feeling of success that I had. In early December 2009, I became a Weight Watchers employee.

Later that month, on December 25, 2009, my mother lost her battle.

But that wasn't when I started binge eating. My binge eating started at about year five of following the Weight Watchers program.

The binge-eating behavior was something completely new to me. I mean, I was pretty good at being in control of pretty much all areas of my life, but suddenly I was losing control around food. I found myself sneak eating everywhere—at home, at parties. The shame of binge eating carried over to all my eating behavior. And thus began the quest to find a solution.

I tried different diets, exercise programs, and supplements to alter my appetite, but those didn't help. No matter what I tried, the binge eating would come back in force.

Finally, I found the Institute for the Psychology of Eating. I enrolled in their certification program, not because I wanted to become a coach but because I was hoping it would help me put my binge eating behind me.

I learned that dieting is a leading predictor of weight gain and a major risk factor in the development of disordered eating. In fact, dieting could itself be considered a form of disordered eating. I also learned that chronic dieting compromises your metabolism and increases the risk of a number of health consequences.

I realized that long-term dieting had not only disconnected me from my body's wisdom but had left me in a nutritionally unbalanced state. I mean, the fact that

I binged on peanut butter? Predictable after following a low-fat diet for many years. The binge eating was my body's way of screaming for attention.

And so began my journey of coming back to myself, of learning to listen to and trust my body once again. Along the way, I learned tools to help me manage my emotions so that I needn't rely on food for that. I learned that there's a lot more to eating than just what we eat. My freedom transformation took me from being a frustrated, fearful, shameful, socially withdrawn binge eater to a confident, balanced woman for whom food is an important component of a healthy life, where health encompasses more than just the physical. It also includes emotional, social, and spiritual health.

I was so profoundly affected by what I learned that I left my job to start my own coaching practice. It is now my privilege to partner with people all across the world in creating their own transformations, through private and group coaching services, courses, and workshops. I've made it my mission to share what I know with as many people as I can so that they can find the peace around food that they so deserve.

And now it's your turn. This book invites you to reconnect with your inner body, using the same tools that I used in my own journey and that I now share with my clients. At the end of each chapter, you'll be challenged by a set of activities that will help you explore and shift your relationship with food. Many of these activities are journaling activities. I invite you to use a nice, attractive, dedicated journal for this work.

I encourage you to engage with the activities fully. After all, transformation doesn't happen just by reading a book.

As I like to say, "What you eat is only part of the story." The rest of the story, the how, when, where, who, and why of eating, is just as important as the what, if not more so. And it's the rest of the story that has been missing from the conversation.

Not anymore.

But before we can address the rest of the story, we have to first talk about letting go.

Two

LETTING GO

I used to weigh myself every day. I'd get up in the morning, go to the bathroom, and then step on the scale first thing. Depending on what the scale said, I would adjust my plans for the day.

Of course, the scale didn't really talk. But in my mind, it kind of did. Some days it would say, "You're doing great. Why don't you treat yourself to a little something special? Or maybe ease up, or even skip, your workout?" Other days it would say, "Boy, you're never going to get this. What the hell did you do? You know you can't stray any one little bit because this is the result. You better put in some extra time at the gym and really watch what you eat to get back on track. Maybe you need to skip lunch today."

During my freedom transformation, I was encouraged to stop weighing myself. I remember hiding the scale in my bathroom closet. But after just a couple days, I found myself sneaking it out. So then I wrapped it up in a towel and put it up on the shelf in my broom closet, far away from the bedroom.

I remember feeling anxious in the morning because I wasn't weighing myself. It felt really weird to not know the number. What was I to do? How was I supposed to navigate my day?

To calm my anxious feeling, I began repeating a little phrase to myself: "I don't know how much I weigh, and you know what? That's OK." I like rhymes.

After a time, I stopped the rhyme and instead began my day with "Good morning, world. What do I get to do today?"

Asking that powerful question made me feel great! It made everything I was going to do that day feel like a privilege, whether my to-do list included work or household chores. By changing my "to do" list to a "get to do" list, my whole outlook on the day shifted for the better.

I let go of my scale routine to make way for a new one that helped me consistently start my day on a positive note. That was my first big step to freedom.

*B*efore you can begin creating a new relationship with food, you need to make some room. You need to let go of things that are no longer serving you so you can invite in new behavior and thought patterns in their place. Just like when you buy new furniture for your living room, you need to clear out the old before you can bring in the new.

What do you need to let go of? Diet mentality.

Diet mentality has become an insidious part of our culture, so much so that we have a hard time recognizing it for what it is. So it's worth spending time looking at what diet culture has done for us and how we can recognize it before we explore how to let it go.

The diet industry—success through failure

The diet industry is a $60-billion-a-year industry with a failure rate of more than 95 percent. Great for them.

They get repeat customers. The success of the diet industry is dependent on our failure! But bad for us because we just keep getting on the dieting hamster wheel, thinking this time will somehow be different (isn't that the definition of insanity?). We do this despite knowing deep down that they don't work.

The fact that diets fail over 95 percent of the time may not be news to you. I mean, you are part of that statistic, as am I. Let's be clear about what we mean by "diet" and "fail," though.

When I talk about dieting, I am talking about the explicit manipulation of food intake (and other behaviors) for the purpose of losing weight. There is a more general definition of "diet" that just means "what I eat." But most people aren't referring to that definition when they use the word "diet" nowadays.

In evaluating a diet's success or failure, it's important to look at the long term. Yes, people who go on diets may experience weight loss. But 95 percent of dieters regain the weight they've lost within a year or two. And when you look longer term, the failure rate is even higher. It is estimated that less than one percent of dieters are able to maintain their weight loss for more than five years, and they often do so at the expense of their own mental wellness, as these "successful" dieters tend to develop obsessive behaviors around food, body, and exercise.

I witnessed diet failure myself during my tenure at Weight Watchers. Most of the members who joined were returning members, back for another round. They'd walk through the door to sign up again, proclaiming, "It worked for me before." Except that it didn't. If it had really worked, they wouldn't need to return. Now I was just as blind to the evidence right in front of me as they were. I wasn't thinking long term either. I was trapped in diet culture, as were they. But now that I have broken free, I can see the hard truth.

Dieting is a major predictor of weight gain, and dieting dramatically increases the risk of developing a clinical eating disorder. Of course, we know that a lot of eating disorders go undiagnosed, as did mine, so the risk is even higher than what the research shows. In fact, the style of eating advocated by many diets could be viewed as a form of disordered eating.

The research is there. This shouldn't be news. We've known for a long time that diets don't work. Yet people continue to be drawn in by the marketing messages: losing weight is easy; thinness is the royal road to happiness. But it just isn't so.

Dieting harms your body physically

Not only do diets not work but they can actually cause harm!

Dieting decreases your metabolism, meaning you burn fewer calories on a regular basis. Dieting also affects the hormones your body uses to regulate hunger. People who have dieted experience an increase in production of the hunger hormone *ghrelin* and a decrease in production of the fullness hormone *leptin*. In other words, dieting makes you hungry more often, and it makes it harder for you to feel satisfied.

No wonder people regain weight. Their metabolisms are slower, and their hormones are driving them to eat. In other words, it is nearly impossible to lose weight and keep it off through dieting. Yet we allow the industry to suggest to us that if it doesn't work, it's somehow our fault. Guess what. You are not a failure for not being a successful dieter. You are just human.

Once the weight gain sets in, what do we do? Go back on a diet—maybe the same one because we tell ourselves it worked before. Or maybe we try something different. And so on. And so on. And that's how we become chronic yo-yo dieters.

Well, more bad news. The weight cycling brought on by chronic yo-yo dieting is associated with cardiovascular disease, blood sugar abnormalities, and increased mortality risk. Interestingly, people who would be classified as overweight or obese but who maintain their weight while engaging in healthy behaviors rather than weight cycling have far lower risk of these conditions.

Diets disconnect you from body wisdom

Dieting has you eat according to a set of external rules—rules that are not based on, well, you. These rules could involve some kind of count (calories, points, or macronutrient grams). They could tell you when you should and shouldn't eat or how many meals and snacks you are allowed to have in a day. The rules may come in the form of portion sizes—including consumption of pre-portioned meals provided by a diet company.

What does this teach you?

It teaches you to eat according to these rules, not according to what your body wants and needs. It teaches you to tune out your hunger and fullness signals so you can accommodate a meal schedule, a certain portion size, a target calorie count, or a specified timing schedule. It teaches you to choose foods based on numbers, or food lists, or rules, not based on how they make you feel. And it teaches you that all bodies should be able to follow the same set of rules and get the desired results.

In contrast, here's what normal eating looks like.

You eat when you're hungry and stop when you feel satisfied—whether it is a traditional mealtime or not and whether it's close to bedtime or not.

You choose foods that make you feel good—ones that give you the energy you need and ones that sustain you until you get hungry again.

You choose foods that nourish you on a physical, emotional, and even spiritual level because you want to take care of yourself.

Any food is a possible food for you. You don't have a list of forbidden foods. There aren't any good foods or bad foods or guilt foods or shameful foods. There are foods you like because they give you pleasure. There are foods you like because they give you energy. And there are foods you don't like because you don't like the way they make you feel. Maybe they make you feel drained and lethargic. Maybe they make you feel ill. You honor your body's reaction and gravitate toward the foods that make you feel the best over time.

This is what a normal eater does most of the time.

Does this sound like a pipe dream? If you've been dieting for a long time, it just might. Part of your healing will involve becoming reconnected to your body and listening to its signals. Don't worry. This book will help you with that.

Morality and food

Speaking of good and bad foods, I want to briefly address this dichotomy. I frequently hear my clients say things like, "I ate something bad," "My eating was really good this week," or "I had a really bad week because I ate a lot of bad foods." When we say such things, we subconsciously judge ourselves as being good or bad. And these judgments are harmful and demoralizing.

Start to notice in your own thoughts and speech whether you talk about food this way. Most people do, so you wouldn't be alone.

And start to tell yourself this:

There are no good foods or bad foods.
There's just food.

Let's remove morality from food. Food is just food. Some foods we like, and some we don't. Some foods make us feel good, and some don't. A food that makes me feel good could make you feel ill. We are unique in that way. But importantly, food itself is not inherently good or bad.

The same is true of music, or exercise, or even something as simple as color. Some we like, and some we don't. Some make us feel good, and some don't. It's not that the music or exercise or color is inherently good or bad. If I don't like country music, spin classes, or the color pink, if those things don't make me feel good, it doesn't make them inherently bad. And I am not a bad person for listening to country music, taking a spin class, or wearing pink on occasion.

When you remove the morality from food, you remove the self-judgment that goes along with that. You also remove the guilt and shame and the spiral of negativity that might follow. Who needs that?

Food is just food. Choose what makes you feel good.

Recognizing the dieter's mind-set

Even though you may have accepted that diets don't work, and even though you believe you have given up dieting, the dieter's mind-set can still be operating in very subtle ways. Here are a few examples of thoughts and behaviors that are representative of a dieter's mind-set.

1. You think of foods as good and bad, or clean and dirty. You have good eating days and bad eating days. Or you think that some days you eat clean and others you don't.
2. You have a list of forbidden foods—ones that are never allowed in your house or that you are never allowed to have.
3. You follow rules about how or when you should eat. Examples: "I need more protein in this meal." "I shouldn't eat after seven at night." "I need to eat because it's lunchtime, even though I'm not really hungry."
4. You find yourself rebelling against your rules of how or when you should eat. Yep, if you find yourself rebelling, then a part of you is still clinging to dieting rules. Otherwise, there'd be nothing to rebel against.
5. You use your willpower to suppress your natural desires. For example, you don't allow yourself to eat when you feel hungry.
6. You follow your hunger and desires, but only up to a certain point because sometimes they're just wrong.
7. You weigh yourself and then, based on that number, make a decision about how you are going to eat or exercise that day.

8. Because you ate "badly" yesterday, you go to the gym and do extra cardio.
9. You have a section in your closet for all the clothes that don't fit you, that you vow you will fit into some day (even though some of them are several years old).
10. You think, "I'm a failure for eating X," or "I'm such a loser for eating Y."
11. You still hold a lingering hope that somewhere out there is that elusive, magical diet that will fix everything, but you just haven't found it yet.
12. You think, "I'll start eating intuitively once I hit my goal weight. That's how I'll maintain my goal weight."

What other thoughts do you have that might be representative of a dieter's mind-set? The activities at the end of this chapter will help you explore them.

Ditch the scale

An important aspect of freeing yourself from struggling with food is examining your relationship with the scale (as well as other external evaluative measures like calorie and step trackers). Are you one of those people who weighs yourself every morning first thing when you wake up, like I used to be? Do you weigh yourself at other times during the day? What are the thoughts that go through your head before and after you step on the scale? Are they at all like these?

- "I'm afraid to look."
- "I knew I shouldn't have had that bagel yesterday!"
- "Woohoo, I'm down. Now I'll have a great day!"
- "Oh man, how can that be? What's wrong with me?"

Is weighing yourself an empowering experience? Or is it a disempowering experience? Are you letting your mood for the day be determined by the number on the scale? And how might that mood affect your choices throughout the day?

Whenever I work with clients, I ask them to not weigh themselves. In fact, I ask them to hide their scales (or have their spouses hide them, or even throw them out). As you read that, what comes up for you? Do you feel trepidation? The best way to find out how the scale affects you is to ditch it!

When I make this suggestion, I typically hear, "But if I don't weigh myself, how will I know what's working and what isn't?"

First, "what's working" depends on what your goal is. I strongly encourage you to let go of the goal of losing weight. Your weight is a side effect of so many things. It's not something you can directly control. When I work with clients, we set goals that do not involve weight—for example, using body wisdom to guide eating decisions, having more energy, sleeping better, feeling less stressful, reducing emotional eating, or creating joyful movement routines. Weight will adjust as a side effect.

Second, notice the belief embedded in that statement: "I need the scale to tell me what's working and what isn't because I can't figure that out by myself." Do you really want to continue to depend on the scale in this way?

Just imagine for a moment a universe in which the scale had never been invented. Sounds heavenly, right? In such a universe, how might we measure progress toward our health goals? Well, we could check in on how we feel. Do we feel more energetic, vibrant, and alive? Are we moving better or differently? Do we notice less pain in our joints? Are we sleeping better? How are our clothes fitting? What do we see when we look in the mirror? Of course, that can be a tricky one because we see ourselves with biased eyes.

In fact, these are all more important measures than a silly number. And why do we elevate that one number in importance? Why is that number so much more important than our blood sugar, blood pressure, or any other measure?

The scale just tells you a number. Don't let an inanimate object determine your mood and your self-worth.

Take back your power.

Ditch your scale.

More thought patterns to let go

While you are in the business of letting go, here are some thought patterns to watch for:

- "I will always struggle with food."
- "I can't have chocolate in the house. I devour it all."

These thoughts give food control over you. Worse, they do so for all time. Your words have power. Your thoughts create your experience. Watch your words, and begin to shift them.

Notice how these feel different:

- "I used to struggle with food, but I'm letting that struggle go."
- "Up until now, I have struggled with food."
- "I used to be someone who mindlessly devoured any chocolate in the house in one sitting, but not anymore."

Watch for patterns that imply "for all time" or "always and forever" and shift those to "up until now" to help you open up to the possibility that things can be different. This will help open your doorway to transformation.

Here's another pattern to watch for:
"I need to have something sweet after dinner."

Notice what happens when you change it like this:
"I enjoy having something sweet after dinner."

You've taken back control. You've turned something that once seemed beyond your control into a choice. Take back your power of choice. When you do so, you might be surprised by the choices you make!

Activities

The activities in this chapter are designed to help you identify and transform your dieter's mind-set. I encourage you to work through them before proceeding to the next chapter.

1. EXPLORING YOUR DIETER'S MIND-SET

The goal of this journaling activity is to build compassionate awareness around how the dieter's mind-set might have a hold on you. It will also help you become aware of your diet thoughts and begin to transform them.

Here's what I'd like you to do:

1. Create a list of some of the ways you hold on to a dieter's mind-set. Use curiosity, not judgment, as you do so. In other words, rather than judging yourself or the thought as bad and admonishing yourself for having such thoughts, try to adopt an approach of "Isn't it interesting that I have this thought?" These thoughts are perfectly understandable in our diet-obsessed culture. Everyone will have some of these thoughts.
2. Acknowledge that these thoughts are an obstacle standing in your way. They are holding you back from stepping into your true self.
3. For each thought in your list, try writing back to it from a nondiet mentality. If it helps, imagine that a friend of yours spoke the thought to you. How might you as a nondieter respond?

For example:

Dieter's thought: "I ate so clean today!"

Nondieter's thought: "Wow, I really felt great today. I ate foods that nourished me and gave me good energy throughout the day. I really like feeling this way!"

Continue this activity as you progress through the course, noticing remnants of the dieter's mind-set and responding to them compassionately from a nondiet perspective.

You may notice resistance come up as you do this exercise—resistance to having these thoughts examined and transformed. If you've been operating from a dieter's mind-set for a long time, this can happen. You may also experience sadness, frustration, or other emotions as you start examining and challenging long-held beliefs. This is understandable.

Do the best you can to practice curiosity and compassion rather than judgment. I have found that it often helps to laugh at yourself. "Ha-ha, there's that silly thought coming up again." And then just let it go.

2. ESTABLISHING NEW THOUGHT PATTERNS
The previous activity helped you explore your dieter thought patterns by identifying them and reframing them into nondieter alternatives. This allows you to practice cognitive flexibility and see that there are other possibilities besides the ways you've been habitually thinking.

Now I want you to work on transforming those thought patterns. The way you do that isn't by not thinking those thoughts; instead, you create new thought patterns that become more prominent. Here's what I'd like you to do.

1. Select one of your dieter's mind-set thought patterns. Start with the one that feels most charged, or most ingrained for you.
2. Examine your rebuttal to that thought pattern and create an affirmation reflecting what you would like to believe instead.
3. Repeat that affirmation five to ten times in a row, multiple times a day. I suggest you set an alarm to go off every hour. Make the alarm message your affirmation. When the alarm goes off, repeat the affirmation to yourself five to ten times.

Here's an example:

Dieter thought: "I've been so good. I deserve to eat this."

Alternative thought and affirmation: "I deserve to eat what I like when I like, unconditionally. Food is just food. It's not something I need to earn."

Work with the same affirmation for one week. Then if you feel you are ready, you can repeat this activity with a new affirmation.

3. CHALLENGE: DITCH YOUR SCALE!
Get rid of it. Hide it—or better yet, throw it out. It doesn't serve you or anyone in your household.

While you're at it, let go of other behaviors that may be reflections of using external measures to judge and evaluate yourself. For example, weighing and measuring your food (except where needed for recipes), tracking food counts (calories, grams, or points), and tracking exercise.

If you have resistance to what you are being asked to do here, don't be surprised! Think of ditching your scale as an experiment. You can always go back to what you were doing before. But won't it be interesting to explore what life is like without it?

4. WHAT HAVE YOU LEARNED?
In your journal, write about what you've learned about yourself and your thought patterns. Based on your insights in this chapter, how would you like to be experiencing life differently six months from now?

Three

IT'S NOT A RACE!

One of the characteristics of binge eating is that it tends to be fast and furious. I remember feeling the need to eat as much as I could as quickly as I could. I would put more food in my mouth before I had even partially chewed what was already there. There were even times when I began to choke. And there certainly was no taste and no pleasure. I guess that's why I was able to eat such junk—taste didn't matter.

I'm not sure why I felt the need to consume so rapidly. Perhaps I wanted to make sure I got a good binge in before I returned to my senses. Or before I got caught.

Would you consider yourself to be a fast eater, a moderate-speed eater, or a slow eater? Most people I ask classify themselves as fast eaters. We rush through each meal as if eating were an inconvenience or a waste of time. We eat on the go, while we're doing things around the house—or even while we're driving.

Ironically, the same people who tell me they rush through their meals usually tell me they absolutely love food. But if you really love food, don't you want to spend some time with it? Isn't that what you do with things you love?

Believe me when I say slowing down when you eat is one of the most significant changes you can make to improve your relationship with food. I have experienced this myself, and I have seen it with my clients. It sounds simple, but it can be quite difficult in practice.

Why is slowing down so important? First, the speed at which you eat can dramatically affect how your body metabolizes the meal. Second, eating slowly is a necessary precursor to all the other practices I'm going to encourage you to explore on your journey to end your food fight.

What eating quickly does to your body

When you eat quickly, you create a stress response in your body. Let's look at just some of the effects of this stress response.

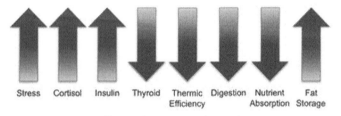

| Stress | Cortisol | Insulin | Thyroid | Thermic Efficiency | Digestion | Nutrient Absorption | Fat Storage |

Effects of Stress on the Body

An increase in stress causes a rise in the level of the stress hormone *cortisol* in your body. You can think of cortisol as one of your body's messengers. Cortisol tells the body's systems, "Hey, there's a stressful situation here. We need to prepare for it." One way the body reacts is by altering blood flow. Blood flow to your limbs and lower brain is prioritized, or increased, under stress. This supports quick physical action and fast, intuitive thinking, which are very helpful when dealing with a stressful situation. In order to increase blood flow to these priority areas, blood flow is routed away from the digestive system and the higher, thinking brain. This means your ability to digest food is diminished, as is your ability to make rational, well-thought-out decisions. Because digestion is impaired, your nutrient absorption goes down. You aren't able to fully absorb the nutrients from the food as it passes through your digestive system. What doesn't get absorbed ends up being excreted instead.

Along with the increase in cortisol levels, the body also produces more insulin. Insulin is the hormone related to blood-sugar regulation. It is also a fat-storing hormone. One of insulin's jobs is to take blood sugar out of the bloodstream and deliver it to the cells that need it. If there's too much sugar in the bloodstream, the insulin will store the excess as fat. If there's not enough blood sugar for the insulin to work on, cravings may soon follow. Having steady blood sugar means having a balanced match between insulin and blood sugar in the bloodstream. When there's a mismatch, one may experience cravings, weight increase, an energy roller coaster, and, over time, insulin resistance.

Chronic stress can also decrease your thyroid output, which decreases your calorie burning, also known as your thermic efficiency or basal metabolic rate.

Finally, when under stress, your body favors storing fat rather than burning it.

Now the stress response can be a wonderful thing when it is used for what it was designed. It was designed to help us deal with a short-term emergency—about three to four minutes long.

The problem is that many of us operate under some degree of stress pretty much all the time. This chronic stress can have some serious consequences for our well-being.

- *Weight gain.* Because chronic stress can decrease your metabolism, even if you keep your food intake and energy expenditure constant, you can end up gaining weight. Also, under stress, your body is in a fat-storing mode, rather than in a fat-burning mode.
- *Increased appetite.* Under stress, your body's digestive system is not operating efficiently, so nutrient absorption is lowered. The way your body reacts to a lack of nutrients is by increasing production of ghrelin, the hunger hormone, in order to try to get you to eat more. In other words, you'll feel hungrier because you are nutrient deprived.
- *Malnutrition.* Over time, poor nutrient absorption can lead to malnutrition. You can be eating the healthiest food on the planet, but if you are under constant stress, you can still be malnourished.
- *Indigestion and heartburn.* Stress triggers changes in the production of digestive juices, swallowing rate, gastric emptying time, and more, all of which can *contribute* to an increase in indigestion and heartburn.

- *Food sensitivities.* Because food is not being digested well, larger particles make it into areas where they can cause *irritation* and damage, leading to the development of food sensitivities.
- *Constipation or diarrhea.* Impaired digestive function can lead to either of these conditions, depending on what is consumed and how the long food stays in the stomach before moving onward through the system.
- *Increased risk of osteoporosis.* As nutrients are not being absorbed well (especially minerals), loss of bone mass is a risk.
- *And more.* Other problems include elevated low-density lipoprotein (LDL) cholesterol, elevated triglycerides, salt retention, destruction of *healthy* gut bacteria, decreased oxygen supply, and decreased kidney function (leading to higher toxicity, water retention, and electrolyte imbalance).

The bottom line is this: eating quickly increases stress. Chronic stress leads to increased hunger and cravings, a stronger likelihood of overeating, weight gain, and other potentially significant health consequences.

But wait. There's more.

Another interesting consequence of stress is that it is incompatible with experiencing pleasure. In other words, if you are stressed out, you'll have a really hard time enjoying your meal. And when your brain doesn't perceive the pleasure and satisfaction of a meal, you will be biologically driven to eat more.

Because stress has such far-reaching consequences, stress management is a major area of focus in my private practice. I use a three-tiered approach to stress management, as laid out in the stress-management pyramid.

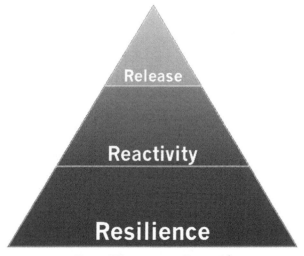

Stress-Management Pyramid

The foundational tier is about building stress *resilience*. The more resilient you are to stress, the less you will be affected by it. Things just won't stress you out as often, or to the same degree.

Reactivity emphasizes changing how you react to situations so that you avoid going into a stress response. Here the work focuses on shifting your mind-set so that situations that once stressed you no longer do so.

The final tier, *release,* acknowledges that stress will happen, but if you can move yourself out of stress and into relaxation quickly, the effect will be short-lived. Below I introduce one *release* technique that you can use to move yourself into a state of relaxation when you sit down to a meal. We'll come back to the topic of stress again in chapter seven, when we talk about eating for reasons other than hunger—that is, when we talk about emotional eating. There we'll dive into the three tiers in more detail.

For now, let's focus on slowing down when you eat. This is an important step in reducing stress—especially stress that may arise in your relationship with food.

Ways to slow down

So how can you slow down with eating? Here are some strategies to experiment with.

1. Take some long, deep breaths before you begin eating. Deep breathing is a great stress-*release* technique that can move you out of stress and

into relaxation, which will empower your digestive system. I recommend what's called a five-five-seven breath: inhale to a count of five, hold for a count of five, and then exhale to a count of seven (or more). What you are aiming to do is hold your breath briefly and then have a nice, long exhale—longer than your inhale. Try this style of deep breathing about five times before your meal, and see how it feels. Bonus: you can use this breathing technique any time you are feeling stressed to help move you into relaxation. This is one of my favorite stress-release techniques. I've gotten into the habit of using it when I'm sitting in traffic at a red light.

2. Chew your food thoroughly. Believe it or not, chewing is one of the most important aids to digestion. Yet most of us barely chew our food at all! We might as well have a tube in our side that says, "Insert food here," and avoids the mouth altogether. But chewing is not only how we taste our food. Chewing plays an important role in helping the digestive system break down and absorb the nutrients in food.

   By chewing your food thoroughly, you will be less likely to suffer from digestive distress. You should aim to have your food be almost liquid before you swallow. Even if you only have five minutes for a meal, let the chewing relax you. Use it almost as a meditation. That way you'll enjoy the whole spectrum of tastes and aromas that make up the meal. And you'll allow your brain and body to be satisfied with having a meal experience, which, as we will see in the next chapter, is also very important for digestion.

3. Put down your utensil between bites. Let it go, and don't pick it up again until you have completely chewed and swallowed your bite.

4. Take a short break, or several short breaks, during your meal. During these breaks, take some deep breaths and check in with your body to see how it's feeling. We'll be talking more about honoring hunger and fullness in a later chapter, but you can get ahead of the game by starting to get into the habit of pausing to check in. Maybe tell yourself you'll take a break every three minutes or when you are a third or two-thirds of the way through. Experiment with intervals or pausing points that feel right to you.

One of the strategies I didn't list, which I have often heard mentioned, is to drink something (like water) between bites. This strategy is somewhat controversial. Some researchers and nutritionists claim doing so can dilute your digestive juices, making digestion more difficult, while others say it's fine. My recommendation is that you continue to do whatever you've been doing in this area and work on incorporating the other strategies to help you slow down. Make the first two—relaxing before you begin eating through breath work and chewing thoroughly—your priority.

If you are used to eating quickly, eating slowly might seem pretty difficult. I want to encourage you to view this as a practice. What you want to try to do is slowly increase the time it takes you to eat your meals. You can even focus on one meal at a time. For example, maybe work on dinner first, then lunch, and then breakfast.

What are you aiming for? Twenty minutes is generally a good amount of time, although the time it takes will depend on the meal size. What you want to aim for is the feeling that you have slowed down to the point where you are chewing thoroughly and swallowing fully before beginning your next bite.

Slowing down will definitely get you well on your way to ending your food fight. But of course, there's a bit more to it than that. Read on to learn about how your mind is a powerful digestive organ and what you can do to take advantage.

Activities

1. PRACTICE SLOWING DOWN
Follow the steps outlined below to begin slowing down when you eat.

1. For a couple of days, just eat the way you normally would, but note how long it takes you to complete your meals. If you want, you can record the information somewhere. Just jot down the start time and end time of your meal, or the duration of your meal, using whatever method feels right for you. You might also want to record the date and what you ate.

2. When you are ready, begin to slowly increase your mealtime. Decide which meal or meals you want to work on, and try to increase your mealtime by five minutes. For example, maybe you want to begin by focusing only on lunch, or you want to practice during particular days of the week. Record your progress in whatever way feels good to you. I also encourage you to journal what techniques you used to slow down, how it felt for you, and any thoughts that came up for you while you were doing it.

3. Once you feel you are comfortable with step two and you are ready to expand your practice, you can either work on increasing the same meal another five minutes or work on a different meal.

It bears worth repeating: this is a practice. You are aiming for progress, not perfection. You are aiming to eat slowly most of the time. Even after practicing slowing down for several years, I still sometimes find myself rushing through. What do I do when this happens? I offer myself some compassion for that experience, and I move on.

2. WHAT HAVE YOU LEARNED?

In your journal, write about what you learned about yourself while practicing slowing down. What was it like for you to slow down? Was it easy or difficult? What influenced your eating speed (e.g., time of day, dining companions, location)? What thoughts did you notice coming up for you as you engaged in this practice?

It is common to notice thoughts of resistance when you start to slow down with your food. Try to note them without judgment. Get curious. Explore with an open mind. Your observations can reveal important insights about your relationship with food. These places are ripe for transformation, and you will have the opportunity to further explore them in later chapters.

Four

BRINGING AWARENESS TO THE TABLE

Why is it so hard to just eat? Why do we feel such a strong need to be doing something else—anything else—whenever we eat? Has eating become such a chore that we'll do anything to make sure we aren't just eating?

One interesting aspect of my binge eating was that it was just eating. There was nothing else going on. But that's because for me, binge eating was an out-of-body experience. I remember the feeling of my mind floating, as if outside my body, helplessly watching me binge from a distance. When the binge was over, my mind would return. There was no awareness, no enjoyment, no real experience at all. Except that physically I would end up stuffed and bloated and yucky and wonder why the hell I did this again.

*H*ave you ever had the experience where you catch a smell of a food, or you walk by a display of food, and you start salivating? Maybe your stomach even starts growling. Or have you ever heard someone say, "Just thinking about or talking about food makes me hungry"? That's your brain performing its digestive function!

Didn't know your brain plays a key role in your digestion? In fact, researchers estimate that 30–40 percent of your total digestive response to any meal is due to what's called the cephalic phase digestive response (CPDR). "Cephalic" means "of or relating to the head." As your brain registers sensations of taste, aroma, satisfaction, or visual stimulation, it initiates secretion of saliva, gastric acid, and enzymes; increases blood flow to the digestive organs; and initiates rhythmic contraction in the stomach and intestines, all to prepare for digestion. Put simply, digestion begins in the head. It begins with awareness of the meal.

What's the most important word in the previous paragraph? "Awareness." Something we rarely bring to the table, as most of the time, we eat while concentrating on something else.

Why is this important?

Your body can be tricked into thinking it is eating by being exposed to food-related thoughts, sights, and smells. You can bet marketers are taking advantage of this fact. That's why the bakery section in the grocery store is always near the front—so you get hit by those smells.

But your body can also be tricked into thinking you're not eating when you actually are. That's what multitasking does.

If you are multitasking while you eat, then you are not fully aware of what you are eating, which means your body is not using its full digestive power.

Think about it: if 30–40 percent of our total digestive response stems from the CPDR—that is, from the head or from awareness—but you multitask while you eat, meaning you're not engaging the CPDR, then you are only digesting at 60–70 percent capacity! You may think, "No big deal. So I don't taste it as much. So what?" Unfortunately, there's more to it than that.

Research has shown that when you eat with distraction, you experience:

- decreased nutrient absorption,
- decreased memory of having had an eating experience, and
- decreased pleasure.

These consequences will all drive up your hunger, leading you to eat more.

Let's look at some of the research.

In one study, test subjects were asked to consume a mineral drink. Absorption was measured in the small intestines for two minerals—sodium and chloride. These minerals were found to be assimilated at 100 percent.

The same subjects were then asked to consume the drink while simultaneously engaging in a listening task. The results indicated a complete shutdown in sodium and chloride assimilation for up to one hour afterward—that is, assimilation went down to 0 percent.

Consuming a simple mineral drink while listening resulted in no nutrient assimilation.

In another study, subjects' digestive activity was measured using electrogastrographic (EGG) methods while watching a short film. Two conditions were compared. In the first, subjects were given a snack to eat before the film, and in the second, subjects were given a snack to eat during the film. Their digestive activity was measured throughout. The results showed that when the snack was eaten before the film, subjects exhibited normal digestive activity. But when the snack was eaten during the film, digestive activity decreased.

If these simple studies show a decrease in digestive capacity, what do you think happens when you eat while driving? Or while working at your desk?

In addition, there's evidence suggesting that your memory of a meal affects your hunger later. But if you eat while you are distracted, you aren't forming memories about the meal. Consequently, you are more likely to get hungry sooner.

If memory affects hunger, then could we manipulate our hunger, and our fullness, by manipulating our memories? A recent study suggests that might be the case. Here's how the study worked.

Researchers took a group of people and, just before lunch, showed them a picture of a bowl of tomato soup. Half saw a bowl with three hundred milliliters of soup, and half saw a bowl with five hundred milliliters of soup. This is about the difference between a cup and a bowl of soup.

Each subject was then led into cubicles where they ate some tomato soup—either the cup or bowl amount—but they couldn't tell how much soup they were eating because the researchers used a special system that could covertly add or remove soup from the bowl without the subject knowing it. Subjects were just told to eat the soup until they reached a special line on their bowl.

Immediately afterward, the subjects who ended up eating larger amounts of soup reported feeling more satiated than those who ate less. When asked again two and three hours later, it was the picture of the soup they saw earlier that mattered more. Those who had seen the bigger bowl of soup felt less hungry, whether or not they had eaten more soup.

While this research is preliminary, it does suggest that our perception and experience of the meal play a key role. But if we aren't aware, if we are multitasking, our perception and experience of the meal are way off.

And along the lines of how you experience the meal, pleasure also plays an important role in your body's digestive capacity. The extent to which a person enjoys her meal has also been shown to affect nutrient absorption. One series of studies showed that when a pleasurable meal was blended and served like a smoothie, subjects absorbed fewer nutrients. It was the exact same food. Only the presentation differed.

If you are multitasking, you aren't paying attention to your meal, and you aren't able to experience the pleasure associated with it. Reduced digestive capacity, again, will lead to an increase in hunger as your body tries to make up for the nutrients it wasn't able to get from the food you ate.

The main takeaway from this discussion is that multitasking while eating has a significant impact on your relationship with food—and not in a good way.

As Marc David, founder of the Institute for the Psychology of Eating, says in his groundbreaking book *The Slow Down Diet* (David 2005, 65), "Metabolizing a meal is like absorbing a conversation. If you were talking with a friend and she didn't pay any attention, you'd walk away feeling incomplete and wishing for more. The essence of your exchange would have been minimally assimilated at best. The same goes with food."

Activities

Your challenge is to practice eating most of your meals without distraction. Just like slowing down, this is a change that will take practice. Work in small steps. Pick a specific meal, or a specific day of the week, and work on eating without distraction for that selected chunk. When you are ready, expand your practice. Remember: the goal is progress, not perfection.

It is natural for resistance to come up. Notice those thoughts, and jot them down in your journal. Are they dieter thoughts? Use the process from chapter three to explore and transform those.

How can you allow yourself to eat with awareness?

- Give yourself permission to step away from work, or take time for yourself, knowing that you will be able to return to whatever you need to in a short while. This is the most important step—and sometimes the hardest.
- Eat sitting down—not on the go.
- Try to make your dining environment a welcoming one. For example, use nice plates and silverware. Make sure the area is free of clutter. Maybe play some soothing background music.
- Take some deep breaths before you eat. This will help you relax into the eating experience.
- As you are eating, try to notice the different flavors and textures of the food. What can you detect? Which textures do you enjoy most? Which smells?

Of course, you are continuing to practice eating slowly too, right?

As you are adding this layer, notice whether eating with awareness helps you slow down or makes you want to speed up. Just get curious, without judgment, and explore what comes up for you in your journal.

Five

WHEN SHOULD YOU EAT?

"It feels good to be hungry."

"It feels good to be hungry."

That's what I used to say to myself when I was dieting. You see, Hunger was the enemy. Hunger drove me to eat, and I needed to not eat so I could change my body. Because my body was wrong. That's what my doctor told me, and that's what society told me.

I tried fighting Hunger. I tried medicating it away through appetite suppressants. But that didn't get me the change I wanted. Then I tried to convince myself, through my mantra, that Hunger was a desirable thing. I thought this would allow me to better tolerate Hunger so that I wouldn't be driven to respond to it. Can you guess what happened? Yep, binge eating. That's one way to avoid Hunger!

I often hear people bemoan, "If only I could control my appetite!" I used to be one of them. But appetite is not meant to be controlled. It is there for a reason. It is your body communicating that there is a need that is not being satisfied.

Part of my recovery from binge eating required transforming my relationship with Hunger. Now as a practicing intuitive eater (and it is a practice), I am much more attentive to my body's hunger and fullness signals. I have released the fear and anxiety around Hunger, and I accept and trust it as part of my body's innate wisdom. For the most part, I eat when I'm hungry and stop when I'm full. I say "for the most part" because I still occasionally eat for emotional reasons. But I know I feel my best when I honor my body and respect its hunger and fullness. And that is my goal: to feel my best.

We are born as intuitive eaters. Babies eat when they are hungry—they cry, and food is provided— and stop when they are full. You can't force a baby to overeat. But along the way, eating becomes more complicated. We learn to ignore our hunger and fullness signals. We end up eating according to a schedule or some set of diet rules. We keep eating until there is no more, whether the amount is appropriate for our bodies or not. We have become so busy and live so much in our heads that we don't notice how our bodies are communicating with us. We don't notice when our bodies are signaling they need food or they've had enough, and even when we do notice, we don't always respond appropriately.

It's time we reconnect with our bodies and once again become the intuitive eaters we were born as. This means paying attention to our hunger and fullness signals and making eating choices that take those signals into account. When we do, questions about when to eat and how much to eat are answered by body wisdom.

Intuitive eating is in direct contrast with what the diet industry has been telling us. In fact, there is no consensus in the diet industry about when you should eat. You may have heard rules like the following:

- Eat three meals a day—no snacking.
- Don't eat after seven pm.
- Eat five times a day "to keep your metabolism going."

Notice that these rules do not refer to your body's needs—just the clock or a number. In other words, these are dieting rules. These are the kinds of rules we'd like to leave behind.

So when should you eat? Well, there's really a simple answer to this question. You should eat when you are hungry. And you should stop eating when you feel satisfied. Sounds simple, but in practice, it can prove to be quite challenging. Don't worry. I've helped many clients learn to honor their hunger and fullness. And I'm going to help you too.

Honoring your hunger

What does honoring your hunger mean? It means recognizing what happens internally in your body as it starts to signal the need for nourishment and honoring that (or trusting that) by making plans to have something to eat.

What someone who honors her hunger *doesn't* do is think:

- "Well, if I can just tough it out a little longer…"
- "That can't be right. I just ate!"
- "But it isn't noon yet!"

- "It's after seven, so I'll just go to bed and tough it out until tomorrow."

Those thoughts are all dieter's mind-set thoughts about when it is appropriate to eat. They also hint at not trusting your body's communication signals. If these thoughts are coming up for you, add them to your list from chapter two, write a rebuttal to transform those thoughts, and then acknowledge them like they are an old, bad penny. Laugh them off, and let them go.

What happens in your body when you start to feel hungry? You may notice an empty feeling in your stomach, your stomach growling, or that you feel light-headed, weak, or tired. If you're one of those people who have difficulty feeling hunger, don't worry—you are not alone. We'll talk about that more in a bit. For now, let's assume you are familiar with how hunger feels in your body and how those feelings change depending on the degree of hunger.

How do you honor hunger? The idea is that instead of waiting until you're so hungry you could eat a horse, you tune in and notice the internal signal that the body needs nourishment.

Think of hunger as being like the gas gauge on your car. When the car is running low on gas, the gas gauge's warning light comes on. You know when that light comes on, you have a bit of a buffer before the tank is completely empty. So you create and execute a plan to refuel your car before you run out completely.

Your body works in a similar way. Your hunger signals are like the low-fuel warning in your car, except hunger signals intensify the longer you go without refueling. And just like with your car, you don't want to wait until you run out of gas to eat. Why? Because that's when the crazy unleashes. Have you ever noticed what happens when you get super hungry? Maybe your eyes glaze over and you slump in your chair, unable to do anything. Or maybe you become a very unpleasant person and take it out on those around you. You may even become light-headed or nauseated.

If you let yourself get too hungry, it's almost impossible to think clearly or make good decisions. The need for energy, the need to address that hunger, becomes so irresistible you'll eat almost anything, whether it provides your body with the nutrients it wants or not.

You'll also find it very difficult to eat slowly and with awareness. The body's desire to refuel, to take care of what it feels is a desperate condition, will be overpowering.

In other words, you'll probably end up (over)eating a lot of convenience foods in a small amount of time. And then afterward, you may still feel unsatisfied because you didn't eat a real meal. The body is still searching for that meal experience, and appetite won't shut down until you've had what feels like a meal. That's why sometimes when we get too hungry—and if we don't have anything prepared and we can't stop to eat normally—the need to eat becomes so strong that we start snacking, and we can't stop. We never get satiated. What we really need to do is sit down and eat a full meal. But we've gone past the point of being able to do that.

So how do we honor our hunger and avoid allowing our bodies to "run out of gas"?

There are three important components to honoring your hunger.

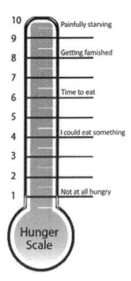

First, you need to be familiar with your hunger warning signals. Take a look at the *hunger scale*. It represents what we know about hunger—the fact that it varies from one extreme of being not in the least bit hungry all the way up to being painfully starving. We experience these hunger levels through a combination of different feelings in our bodies.

Take a look at the scale, and see if you can imagine what it would feel like to be at these different levels. Ask yourself, for example, "How does my body feel when I'm at the 'I could eat something' stage? And how is that different from the 'time to eat' stage?"

In fact, check in with your body right now. Take a deep breath, let it out, and then turn your attention inward. Ask your body, "How hungry are you, on a scale of one to ten?" and see what answer comes forward for you.

Of course, this scale is impressionistic, and there's no right or wrong here. But the scale has proven to be very useful in helping people tune in, notice, and feel their differing hunger levels.

So that's the first step: understanding what your hunger levels are.

Second, you need to check in with your body regularly to see where you're at. Just like you check your gas gauge regularly to make sure you have enough fuel to get where you want to go, you want to check in with your body regularly see where it's at. You can ask your body the same question we did above: "How hungry are you, on a scale of one to ten?" Or maybe ask, "What does my body need right now?" Be open to whatever answer comes up—food, water, a stretch, some movement, or something else entirely.

Checking in with your body regularly in this way can actually be quite challenging, especially given our busy lifestyles. What I hear a lot is, "I just keep going and going, and before I know it, I'm famished." This can easily happen when a person is so busy "in her head" that she doesn't check in with her body at all until it's too late. The body might be screaming for nourishment (or water, or a bathroom break), but no one is listening. If this describes you to some degree, don't worry. One of the activities at the end of this chapter will help you practice checking in regularly.

So once you are familiar with how hunger expresses itself in your body, and you are checking in regularly to notice where you are at, the third step is to act on your hunger appropriately. What I encourage you to do is to try to eat when you are within a four and a six on the hunger scale. Around three or four is when you should start planning your next meal or snack. You want to try to avoid waiting until your hunger is above seven.

Honoring your fullness

Honoring your fullness means eating to the point where your body says, "Ah, I'm good." That's the point where your body is feeling satisfied and energized, where eating more would lead it into feeling too full, lethargic, or worse.

Honoring fullness can be quite challenging for a variety of reasons:

- People with a history of dieting may still be operating, even if subconsciously, under diet rules dictating how much they should or should not be eating. Examples of rules around food amounts include, "The protein portion should be about the size of the palm of the hand," or "You should have no more than a fist-sized amount of pasta." Basically, whenever the word "should" enters the conversation, you should take a second look and ask, "Is this a dieter's 'should'?"
- Because dieters have trained themselves to eat controlled portions, they may not allow themselves to eat enough food to reach the point of satisfaction. Or they may habitually eat beyond it because the portions they've been told to eat are actually too large for them.
- Chronic dieters who have oscillated between being famished and overfull—the hunger or fullness extremes—may find it difficult to sense

intermediate points, such as the satisfaction point, especially when beginning to transition into eating intuitively. But that will change over time through practicing the activities in this book.

- Many have that old "clean your plate" song playing in your head, that song that forces you to finish everything, even if doing so takes you beyond the point of satisfaction.

- Finally, there may be limiting beliefs or fears around food scarcity—of not having enough—that lead you to eat whatever you can when presented with the opportunity.

Nonetheless, whatever your past experience with honoring your fullness, know that from this point onward, things can and will be different. Trust in your body's wisdom, and trust that there is no right or wrong, no pass or fail, in this process. Everything is a learning experience.

I want to share some tools and strategies to help you practice honoring your fullness.

Your first tool is the *fullness scale.* Just as with the hunger scale, it can be helpful to think of fullness in these terms. The descriptions on this scale can help you tune in to how the different levels of fullness might feel in your body.

Notice the scale ranges from "empty," at one, all the way up to feeling so full that you are "sick," at ten. What you are aiming for is to stop eating when you are around four to six on the scale—that is, when you are feeling somewhere between "satisfied: good to go" and "comfortably full." You want to avoid getting above a seven, if you can. That is, you want to avoid getting into the "uncomfortable" or higher range.

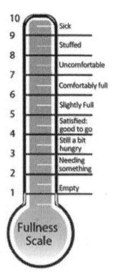

The process for honoring fullness is similar to the one for honoring hunger.

1. Learn what your body feels like when you hit that four to six on the scale.
2. Check in regularly so that you notice when this happens.
3. When you notice that you are satisfied, discontinue eating.

Now I don't know about you, but honoring fullness has been more challenging for me than honoring hunger. That's why I'm spending a little bit more time and detail on it here. Let's look at some strategies that may help:

- In order to learn what your body feels like at the four-to-six fullness level, you may need to experiment with what it feels like to be at other points on the scale. Allow yourself to experiment with stopping at three, or at seven, and learn what that feels like in your body. That can help you define your four-to-six "sweet spot."

- Eating slowly and with awareness (chapters three and four) are key to honoring your fullness. If you eat quickly while distracted, you will have little hope of noticing your fullness level. Frequent check-ins will be necessary. With practice, these check-ins, and stopping at the appropriate point, will become automatic.

- Give yourself permission to stop eating before you've finished everything on your plate. Allow yourself to release your membership in the "clean your plate club," as it no longer serves you.

- Pause throughout your meal, and ask yourself, "If I were to stop now, would I be OK until the next eating opportunity?" If the answer is yes, then stop.

- Make a physical gesture that your meal is complete by pushing your plate away, putting a napkin over it, crossing your silverware over it, or clearing it from the table. This represents an acknowledgment that you decided you were satisfied and can help you resist continuing to pick at your plate as it sits in front of you.

- Declare out loud, to yourself or whomever you are eating with, that you are full. Again, this is acknowledging that your body has reached this point.

Remember: as you are experimenting with your fullness levels, you can always eat again later when you get hungry because you are also honoring your hunger. So it's OK to play around with stopping at a fullness of three, for example, to see how that feels.

Your activities for this chapter encourage you to explore using these strategies as you practice honoring your fullness.

Honoring hunger and fullness is not a dieting rule

The idea of honoring your hunger and fullness is not to be interpreted as a dieting rule, where you are in compliance or not in compliance. Think of them as intuitive-eating practices. Like other practices (e.g., yoga, meditation, slowing down when you eat, eating with awareness), some days will feel better than others, and some days will feel more challenging than others, but you maintain the intention of honoring the practice.

In particular, honoring your hunger does not mean you're *only* allowed to eat when you are physically hungry.

And honoring your fullness does *not* mean you are a failure if you eat beyond the point of satisfaction.

There are a number of situations where you will want to give yourself permission to eat at different levels of hunger and fullness.

- *Preemptive eating.* There may be days when your schedule makes it difficult for you to eat at the time that your body normally enjoys, so for practical reasons, you eat an early lunch before you are meal hungry, or you have an extra snack. You may not be waiting until you are a four to six on the hunger scale, but it is good self-care to notice and act upon challenges in your schedule.
- *Celebrations and social eating.* Many events include special celebratory or traditional foods. Enjoying these foods is an important part of an intuitive-eating lifestyle. Having an empowered and peaceful relationship with food includes allowing yourself to bond and connect through food. You may find yourself eating these foods even though you aren't hungry. Give yourself permission to do so. But do so mindfully, with enjoyment!
- *Eating for pleasure.* Let's face it. Food is pleasurable. If it wasn't, we'd probably rarely eat at all. Sometimes we eat past fullness because we want to continue a pleasurable food experience. An intuitive eater allows herself to experience pleasure

from food. In fact, it's very important to her! But at the same time, she doesn't use food as her sole source of pleasure. If you feel you are relying on food too much as a source of pleasure, for now, just try to be attentive to where you end up on the fullness scale. We'll be returning to this topic in the chapter that addresses emotional eating.

- *Emotional eating.* Eating for emotional reasons, again, is a natural and effective way of managing difficult emotions. We will be addressing emotional eating in more detail in a later chapter. For now, if you are eating emotionally, just notice where you are on the hunger and fullness scales when you start and stop. What emotions or situations trigger emotional eating for you? Note them in your journal, so we can return to them later.

What if I don't feel hunger or fullness?

Your body signals hunger and fullness by releasing hormones into your system. Think of these hormones as little messengers between your brain and your body that communicate nourishment needs.

Just like other hormones (such as insulin or cortisol), your hunger and fullness hormones can get "out of whack." Conditions that can throw off your body's production of hunger and fullness hormones include chronic dieting, weight cycling, stress, lack of sleep, and digestive problems. Research shows that people who have lost weight through calorie-restricting diets have experienced increased production of the hunger hormone ghrelin and decreased production of the fullness hormone leptin. In other words, dieting can affect your hormones so that you are hungry more often and have difficulty feeling satisfied.

You may also have trouble noticing your hunger and fullness signals because you have become used to eating according to dieting rules—rules that have you ignore your body's needs and eat according to a specific schedule and portion size. As a consequence of following these kinds of rules, you may have learned to tune out your body's hunger and fullness signals. In other words, you've turned the volume way down on your hunger-and-fullness radio station—or you've shut the radio off entirely.

This kind of detachment from body feedback is also common in people who have suffered through eating disorders like anorexia or bulimia.

People who have engaged in chronic overeating can develop a condition called leptin resistance, which is when the body becomes resistant to the satiation hormone leptin (just like the body can become resistant to insulin, leading to type 2 diabetes).

The good news is that the practices you've been working on—slowing down and eating with awareness, plus the ones in this chapter—will help you reconnect with your hunger and fullness signals. Perhaps you've noticed a difference already. But you may need to be extra patient with yourself, depending on where you are starting from.

Note: If you believe you have leptin resistance or you are having extreme difficulty noticing hunger and fullness, I encourage you to contact me to discuss options to help with this.

Maybe I'm just thirsty

Have you heard this one? "Maybe I'm not hungry at all. Maybe I'm just thirsty."

The signals for hunger and thirst do share some characteristics, but they are not identical. Thirst, or dehydration, generally does not manifest as a grumbling in the stomach. A growling stomach is a sign of physical hunger. However, symptoms of dehydration do include sluggishness, headache, dizziness, and more—and these same symptoms can also accompany the higher levels on the hunger scale.

If you are experiencing these symptoms and you think you might be thirsty, by all means, drink some water. If you feel your stomach grumbling ten to fifteen minutes later, that's a sign of physical hunger. Check in and see where you are on the hunger scale, and honor it the best you can.

Summary

The questions of when and how much to eat are best answered by our body wisdom, specifically, our hunger and fullness signals. The challenge, then, is to get better at listening for, trusting, and acting on those signals. The three-step process introduced in this chapter is designed to help you do just that.

The first step is to learn how different levels of hunger and fullness feel in your body. The hunger and fullness scales are provided as guides to help you with this.

The second step is to get into the habit of checking in with your body regularly. Have a conversation with it. Ask it some questions: "How hungry are you? What do you need? Are you good for now? Have you had enough?" As you build this habit and create a stronger connection with your body, the communication will happen effortlessly.

The third step is to respect your body's hunger and fullness signals by taking appropriate action, that is, by having something to eat or by ceasing to eat. For both hunger and fullness, you are targeting the midrange of the scales. You are aiming to eat when you are at a four to a six on the hunger scale and stop when you are at a four to a six on the fullness scale.

Activities

Your activities are designed to help you practice honoring your hunger and fullness. There are four in all. I suggest you focus on one activity at a time. Work on that activity for a few days, a week, or whatever time frame feels right to you before progressing to the next one. In other words, you may want to take several weeks to complete the activities in this chapter. Give yourself permission to do so.

The fourth activity provides you with some journaling prompts to help you look for patterns in how you observe your hunger and fullness. You can begin to engage in this journaling activity at any time while you are performing the monitoring activities.

1. CHECK IN WITH YOUR BODY REGULARLY

If you feel disconnected from your hunger and fullness signals, I encourage you to start by checking in with your body regularly. You can set a "check-in" alarm to go off a few times during the day (maybe every two hours). Each time the alarm goes off,

1. take one or two deep, cleansing breaths,
2. turn your attention inward, and ask yourself, "In this moment, what am I feeling in my body?"
3. scan your body from head to toe, looking for any feelings of tension, relaxation, aches, warmth, cold, or any sensations whatsoever; and
4. finally, ask yourself, "What might my body need in this moment?" For example, does it need to stretch, move, rest, eat, or drink?

2. HONOR HUNGER LEVELS

Before each meal or snack, rate your hunger level according to the hunger scale (one to ten). Use paper or a spreadsheet to track your observations. You may choose to also record the time of day, what you are eating, and how you are feeling. Record whatever information feels right to you.

Note: if you find tracking like this to be triggering in any way (because you have been involved in excessive tracking as part of your dieting history), skip it! Simply check in with your hunger before you eat.

Ask yourself: Am I at a four-to-six on the hunger scale?

If you notice you are eating too soon, that is, you aren't quite at a four on the hunger scale, what might you do to allow yourself to wait a little longer next time? If you allowed yourself to get too hungry (you have gone beyond a six), what might you do to try to eat a little sooner?

Most importantly, try to avoid judging yourself. You are learning to attune to your body. There will be times when you begin eating outside the four-to-six range. That's important feedback to help grow your understanding of and connection with your body.

3. HONOR FULLNESS LEVELS
Explore honoring your fullness levels using the same process as described in the previous activity.

Remember: no judgment!

4. JOURNAL: WHAT DO YOU NOTICE?
Look over your work for the previous two exercises, and explore the following questions in your journal.

Do you notice any patterns with your *hunger* levels? How soon after a meal or snack do you generally start to experience low or moderate levels of hunger? Is it regular, or does it vary—by day or by previous meal? What might you be able to conclude?

What patterns do you notice about your *fullness* levels? How long does it take you to feel some degree of fullness?

Do you notice any difference in your level of fullness based on how hungry you were when you started eating?

How does fullness feel in your body? Are you able to notice different fullness levels?

Do you notice any differences in fullness levels based on the types of foods you eat?

What thoughts, judgments, or emotions come up for you as you are tracking your hunger and fullness?

What thoughts, judgments, fears, or other emotions come up for you as you are trying to stop eating based on your fullness level? Might any of those represent dieter's mind-set (or other rule-based) beliefs? If so, go back to the "establishing new thought patterns" activity in chapter two and work on transforming those beliefs.

If you have difficulty stopping before you reach a point of uncomfortable fullness, explore whether any of these factors might be influencing you:

- Restrictive eating earlier in the day.
- Rebelling against what feels like a dieter's mind-set.
- Values or rules around finishing food, allowing leftovers, and so on.
- Emotional eating. (We'll be addressing this later. For now just note it, and allow yourself to be OK with it.)

Remember: honoring your hunger and fullness are not "rules" that we are looking to comply with perfectly. Rather, they are principles that describe how intuitive eaters eat, for the most part. It is natural for intuitive eaters to sometimes eat when they are not hungry and to sometimes eat beyond the point of satisfaction, even into discomfort. However, for the most part, they honor their hunger and fullness.

If you are still feeling like you have work to do in this area, don't be surprised! It definitely takes practice. Be patient with yourself, have compassion, and trust that you are on the right path. Give yourself permission to take the time you deserve to eat mindfully, to check in, and to experiment with what it feels like to eat at different levels of hunger and fullness.

Six

WHO DO YOU INVITE TO THE TABLE?

During my yo-yo diet and binge cycle, the very act of eating felt like going to battle. Food was my enemy. I would sit down to an eating experience filled with stress and confusion. My head would be swimming with thoughts like "Will this make me gain weight? Will I be able to control myself? What will other people think about what I'm eating? Or how I'm eating? Are there too many grams of fat in this meal? Not enough protein? Too many carbs? Please don't order an appetizer! I don't want to be tempted or have to sit and watch others eat it. And take the bread away! If I don't finish this, will I get hungry later and be more likely to binge? I know I shouldn't finish it. Oh, but it tastes so good, and I may never have the chance to experience this again!"

No wonder I was exhausted and drained and just ready to throw in the towel.

In this chapter, we explore the question, "Who are you as an eater?" That is, what kinds of thoughts, beliefs, and emotions do you bring to the table?

Take a moment now and imagine yourself sitting down to a meal. Maybe it's dinner at home, or lunch at work. What are some of the thoughts that go through your head? How do those thoughts change depending on who you are with, where you are, and what the situation is?

Do your thoughts resemble these?

- "Food is the enemy."
- "Ugh, I hate that I have to eat at all."
- "I shouldn't be eating this!"
- "This is going to make me fat!"
- "Why am I eating this? I'm such a willpower weakling!"

Do you tend to think about stressful things while you eat, such as work challenges, finances, or the news?

For people who have experienced an embattled relationship with food and body, the very act of eating itself can be stressful.

This often shows up when you try to slow down when you eat. Slowing down provides space for all those negative, uncomfortable thoughts to surface. If you've been in a constant long-term battle with food, if you feel that food is the enemy, the very act of sitting down to eat is like starting a fight—again!

Why is this important? Well, your mind is extremely powerful. Your thoughts create your experience, including your eating experience. Your thoughts influence your digestion and your appetite. By changing your thoughts, you can significantly shift your relationship with food and body in a profound way.

Your thoughts influence digestion

How can your thoughts influence your digestion? Well, your very thoughts can trigger a stress response. We've talked about the debilitating effects of stress before— how it hinders digestion and nutrient absorption, for example. And we've talked about how stress can be triggered by eating quickly. Well, a stress response can also be triggered by your thoughts.

Consider this definition of stress:

Stress is any threat, real or imagined,
and the body's response to it.

Importantly, your brain doesn't know the difference between a real threat and an imagined one.

You can trigger a stress response just by thinking. You've probably done this before. You're sitting at home, relaxing peacefully, when a thought pops up in your head. You latch onto it and start pursuing it, and it leads to worry and anxiety. All of a sudden, you aren't feeling so good any more. Your breathing becomes shallower and more rapid. Maybe you start to get a little jittery. You aren't thinking as clearly. You feel the need to "fight, flee, or freeze" in some fashion. That's a stress response.

If you've developed a love-hate relationship with food, or perhaps mostly a hate one, the act of eating itself may be a recurring stressful event.

Or if you are in the habit of using mealtime as the time to revisit all the stressful things in your life, you are making your meal a stressful event.

Now one thing we know about stress is that it narrows your reasoning ability—that is, your ability to be deliberate and focused. You have more difficulty eating slowly and attentively. It's harder to notice your fullness or satiety point. And you are less likely to make informed food decisions. In other words, you are more likely to stress-eat.

Yeah, I know. Stress is a big deal. It's entered the discussion a few times. And it will show up again in our next chapter, which focuses on emotional eating. For now, let's focus on the thoughts you bring to the table and how you can shift those thoughts so that you can become a relaxed, peaceful eater. How do you do this?

Five steps to becoming a relaxed eater

1. Before eating, take two to five deep, cleansing breaths. I encourage clients to practice a five-five-seven breath, which means breathe in to a count of five, hold your breath to a count of five, and exhale to a count of seven (or more). By doing so, you will help your body move into a state of relaxation.
2. Express gratitude for the food you are about to consume, either silently or out loud. Perhaps give thanks to those who contributed to you having that food. Offer a prayer. Whatever feels right to you. Why do this? While negative thoughts

produce stress and narrow your thinking, positive thoughts—about love and gratitude, for example—evoke relaxation and can expand your reasoning ability.

3. Express that you are open to receiving the nourishing properties of the food, either aloud or silently. For example, "I am grateful this food will nourish me in body, mind, and spirit."

4. Think about how satisfying the meal will be. You have a choice. You can look at your meal and think, "This won't sustain me at all." Or you can look at the meal and think, "Wow, this is really going to nourish and energize me!"

5. Then proceed to eat your meal slowly and attentively so that you consciously and thoughtfully encode this meal experience into your memory.

You'll get to explore this practice when you work on this chapter's activities. Before you do, though, I'd like to address one particular pattern of thoughts that is so prevalent in our society, and that's the classification of foods into good versus bad.

Good foods and bad foods

I know we've talked about good and bad foods already in the chapter on letting go of your dieter's mind-set. Now is a good time to revisit this, especially because we have a bit more wisdom under our belts.

Here's what's interesting about the idea of good and bad foods (also clean versus unclean foods). As we've seen, the metabolic power of a food is profoundly affected by factors that are not actually part of that food at all! Factors like stress, relaxation, awareness, and even pleasure have significant impacts on how our bodies assimilate food.

Now it's true that certain foods can enhance your physical health, while others might detract from it. And which foods do which is subject to individual variation. But there's no such thing as good or bad foods, particularly in the sense of morally good or morally bad. There's no morality in food.

Consider this analogy. A knife is not good or bad. Similarly, a food isn't good or bad. It all depends on the context. But if you choose to label either of these objects as bad, by extension, you end up labeling yourself as bad for using them. You actually become both the guilty party and the judge.

Worse, when you label a food as good or bad, you close the door on curiosity and discovery. For example, imagine you were told that your new coworker was a real jerk and was only hired because he's related to the boss. What would happen? Well, now he's labeled. The way you approach him, if at all, will be colored by that information, that judgment. You'll stop asking certain questions, and you'll interpret things through the lens of that label.

The same goes with food. Is all sugar bad? Is all white flour bad? What if I combine sugar with other foods—can that change the effect? What if I have just a little? What about alcohol? Is wine good or bad? It all depends on how you use it, right?

But if we close the door on curiosity, we don't explore these questions. We don't tune in to how our bodies enjoy or do not enjoy certain foods. And that disempowers us.

Rather than labeling foods as good or bad (clean or unclean, and so on), rather than judging both the food and yourself, I encourage you to release those thoughts and allow yourself to open up and explore how different foods, in different combinations, affect your body. You'll get to do this in chapter eight when we explore the "what" of eating. By allowing yourself to be an explorer, to be curious, you get to zone in on the foods that make you feel your best, and the question of good or bad goes away. Or better, it evolves into, "What do I like, and what do I dislike?" and "What will feel really good in my body right now?" When you ask those questions, you naturally gravitate toward those foods that are healthiest for your body.

The placebo effect

This may seem a bit of a digression, but I want to emphasize that the mind is truly powerful. I'm sure you've heard of the placebo effect. It's when, for example, you tell someone you're giving her a medication for pain, but you're actually giving her a water pill—and yet she reports that her pain goes away. It's actually estimated that 35–45 percent of all prescription drugs may owe their effectiveness to the placebo effect, and the percentage is even higher for over-the-counter medications.

In one very powerful study from 1983, researchers were testing a new chemotherapy treatment on patients. One group received the actual drug, while another group received a placebo. Both groups were told they were receiving the test drug and what the possible side effects might be. Of the group that received the real drug, 74 percent lost their hair. Astoundingly, of the group that received the placebo, 31 percent lost their hair!

As Marc David observes (David 2005, 125), "If the power of the mind is strong enough to make our hair fall out when taking a placebo, what do you think happens when we think to ourselves: 'This cake is fattening…'?"

I think I'll leave you with that thought and let you take that with you as you explore the activities for this chapter.

Activities

1. EXPLORING YOUR HISTORY AS AN EATER

Journal your history as an eater. Who have you been as an eater at different stages of your life? What thoughts and beliefs have you brought to the table at those different times?

Consider different ages, different diets you may have been on, and different places you've lived and worked and how these things influenced you as an eater.

One way to approach this activity is to imagine yourself at different ages sitting down to a meal. Then journal the experience. Where are you? Who is with you? What are your thoughts and attitudes about food? About the eating experience?

Once you've explored your history, write about how your thoughts and beliefs around food have changed and evolved over time.

Finally, journal where you would like your thoughts and beliefs to go from here.

2. Practice being a relaxed eater

Use the five-step process outlined in this chapter to practice being a relaxed eater. What do you notice? What thoughts come up for you? How do these practices affect your thoughts and feelings about the eating experience?

3. Transform negative thoughts about food

If you've noticed that you have negative thoughts about food, whether during mealtime or at other times, this is the activity for you. Let's work on letting go of those thoughts and replacing them with more positive ones, just as we have done with dieter thoughts.

Create a list of your disempowering or negative food thoughts. Include any thoughts about "good foods" and "bad foods," any "should" and "should not" thoughts, and any worries and stresses about food, food scarcity, missing out, whatever comes to mind for you.

Acknowledge that these thoughts are obstacles standing in your way. They are holding you back from stepping into your true self.

For each thought in your list, try writing back to them from a positive perspective.

For example, "Food is the enemy!"

New perspective: "Food nourishes my body and gives me the energy to do the things I like to do. I am grateful for food and the way it nourishes me."

4. WHAT HAVE YOU LEARNED?

In your journal, write about what you learned about yourself, about who you are as an eater, and about who you would like to be.

Seven

EATING FOR REASONS OTHER THAN HUNGER

During my binge-eating recovery, I very distinctly remember a moment that forever changed me. I was walking through my neighborhood listening to a podcast, just as I had done many, many times before. The sun was shining brightly. I could feel the warmth of it on my skin. I remember exactly where I was, the corner where I was walking, the house I was passing by, when I was suddenly overcome with an overwhelming feeling of grief. I could feel the tears start to run down my face.

Where was this coming from? Why was I feeling this? Why now?

I understood pretty quickly what the grief was about. It was about my mother, who had passed away about five years prior.

And I realized in that moment that I had a choice. I could cut the feeling off. I mean, hadn't I grieved enough already? Or I could open myself up to it and let it flow through me, freely.

For perhaps the first time, I chose the latter. I opened up even more. I began sobbing. As I was almost doubled over in tears, I realized something: the fact that I was able to feel so strongly was a gift! Oh, how amazing, that I could be affected in this way, that I was able to experience such a deep connection that would lead to this grief. Not everyone gets to experience that!

This feeling was not something to be suppressed, but to be embraced!

And as soon as I came to that understanding, where I was able to see my negative emotion in a positive light, my grief was replaced with joy.

*M*any of us are discouraged from overtly expressing emotion. This programming starts at an early age. We are told things like, "Don't cry," "Don't be angry," and "Stop being that way." We internalize the idea that expressing emotions is harmful or burdensome to other people. And so we try to keep them to ourselves as best we can.

Food is a very effective tool for helping us bottle up our emotions. Food has a way of making us feel different from whatever emotion we want to suppress. Large amounts of food can force our bodies into a state of relaxation and lethargy so that we don't feel much of anything. In other words, emotional eating is actually an effective strategy for suppressing emotions.

But emotions aren't meant to be suppressed. Emotions are energy in motion (e-motion). Emotions are meant to move through us. By suppressing them, we are keeping that energy stuck in our bodies. Over time, that stuck energy can lead to dis-ease—both physical and emotional.

While acknowledging that eating is an effective tool for helping us manage our emotions, in this chapter, we'll explore other ways to manage them so that we don't have to rely on food so much.

Everyone is an emotional eater

It is perfectly natural to eat for reasons other than hunger—that is, to eat for what we often label as emotional reasons: pleasure, comfort, distraction, sedation, numbing, to name a few. We may eat when we feel sad, bored, lonely, stressed, happy, or celebratory. As far as I can tell, pretty much any emotion can be associated with eating.

If you have ever described yourself as an emotional eater, know that you are not alone. In fact, everyone is an emotional eater to some degree. The challenge comes when you get into the habit of using food as your primary tool for dealing with uncomfortable feelings and situations.

To start, let's agree that the goal is not to eliminate emotional eating entirely (although many a client has said to me, "I don't want to ever emotionally eat again"). Instead, the goal is to reduce the need to use food for managing emotions.

How do we do that?

1. We're going to give you more tools for your toolbox so that food isn't the only one—or isn't the primary one—available to you.

2. We're going to strengthen your ability to move your emotional energy so that you don't need to turn to a tool to manage your emotions.

3. We'll begin the work of transforming the beliefs and thoughts—the mind-set—that triggers the uncomfortable, intolerable feelings you've been using food to avoid. While we'll be able to bring awareness to those thought patterns, the deeper transformative work is often best addressed through private work with a coach, counselor, or other qualified healer.

You may have already noticed some shifts in your emotional eating behavior as a result of your work on the activities of the previous chapters: slowing down, eating with awareness, attending to hunger and fullness, and being a relaxed and grateful eater. All those practices, wherever you are at with them at this stage, can shift your emotional eating. Why? Because emotional eating tends to have the opposite characteristics: it occurs quickly, mindlessly, independent of hunger and fullness, and not from the perspective of a relaxed and grateful eater. All these practices you've been working on contribute to you having a more mindful, peaceful relationship with food, one in which emotional eating is relegated to a less frequent occurrence.

But these practices alone may not be enough. They weren't enough for me. In this chapter, we'll focus on tools and techniques to help you understand and transform your emotional eating. Specifically, we'll explore the following:

- Is it really emotional eating?
- Are you reacting out of deprivation?
- Is it stress eating?
- If it is emotional eating, how can you identify your emotional eating triggers and explore other (nonfood) ways to move your emotional energy?

Is it really emotional eating?

A lot of people self-diagnose as being emotional overeaters or binge eaters because they watch themselves eating excessively, usually in the late afternoon or after dinner. They feel like they have no control over their eating behavior, that they are compelled to overeat, and they just can't stop. I know exactly what that feels like because I've been there.

However, the compulsion to overeat may not actually stem from emotional reasons. Compulsive overeating can arise due to physical factors like lack of sleep and lack of proper nutrition. Either of these will lead your body to increase hunger to the point where you feel like you have an insatiable need to eat.

If you are not getting the sleep your body needs, I strongly urge you to address this. Sleep is when your body detoxes, repairs, and replenishes itself. Without this, you will feel groggy and lethargic. Your body will produce more hunger hormones, and your hunger will become harder to resist as the day progresses. Insufficient sleep is a stress on your body. It weakens your immunity and makes it difficult to think clearly, meaning you won't make the decisions that are in the best interest of your long-term health.

This is not a book about improving sleep. But if you need help in this area, you can reach out to me or seek help from a professional who specializes in sleep.

Similarly, if your body is not getting the nutrients it needs, it will drive up your hunger. Nutrient deficiencies can arise from:

- Chronic stress. As we've discussed already, stress decreases nutrient absorption, which can lead to malnutrition plus increased appetite.
- Not eating enough food.
- Not getting enough variety in the foods that you are eating.
- Consuming a significant amount of *anti-nutrients*—foods that provide calories but little in the way of vitamins, minerals, and other essentials.

You might want to consider taking some high-quality supplements. The reality is that our food supply is not what it used to be, and it's difficult to get all the nutrients you need from eating whole foods, so a high-quality supplement program is essential. Unfortunately, the market is flooded with low-quality supplements. So do your research to find ones that are highly absorbable and effective.

The next chapter addresses the topic of nutrition in more detail, so I don't want to get deep into that here. But I do want to mention a pattern that I've seen quite frequently: people who eat very little during the day end up binge eating at night.

More specifically, people who are in the habit of eating diet-style or calorie-restricted breakfast, lunch, and snacks (think Special K and skim milk) aren't getting the nutrients their bodies need. What I see commonly in the eating habits of recovering dieters is a lack of healthy essential fatty acids in their food intake. This pattern arises because diets have traditionally emphasized eating very little fat. For some people I've worked with, just adding some healthy fat back, especially early in the day, has reduced their need to binge at night.

In the next chapter, we'll talk more about the "what" of eating. For now, you can take a look at your eating habits and ask yourself,

- "Do most of my meals and snacks have a balance of proteins, healthy fats, and carbohydrates?"
- "Am I allowing myself to eat when I am hungry during the day?"
- "Have I recently experienced a change (in physical activity, medications, and so on) that could affect my hunger?"

Your answers to these questions can point you to where you might experiment with some changes to see how your late-day eating shifts.

Are you reacting out of deprivation?

Is there still a part of you that classifies food in terms of good and bad? Do you feel that certain foods are absolutely off limits? Perhaps there's a part of you that thinks certain foods are only OK at certain times (on vacation, for special celebrations, or only once a month). If so, then you may still be operating from a place of deprivation, and deprivation increases the risk of overeating. These are all diet mentality memes. If you are still struggling in this area, that's OK. It just means you have a little more work to do. Remember, it takes patience, awareness, and practice to release these old beliefs that have been with you for a very long time and build new ones in their place.

You may also feel deprived if your access to food is limited in some way. Perhaps your access is controlled by someone else. If there are people in your life who are judgmental about your food choices, you may feel you have to eat a certain way when you are around them. If you don't feel free to choose what you want without facing backlash, that's a form of deprivation. If this is the case, I suggest you commit to addressing the situation.

Stress eating

Many people turn to food when they are feeling stressed. Recall that your body's stress response (the biochemical reaction that happens in the body under stress) has a number of physiological consequences. While under stress, digestion is inhibited, your metabolism slows, your body favors storing fat, and higher deductive reasoning can be impaired, among other things. Reduced digestion leads to poor nutrient absorption, which means your body needs more food to get the nutrients it needs, so it drives up your appetite. Basically, it's not good. And it gets worse over time.

Beyond the effect of stress on your appetite, it turns out that eating can actually reduce stress in a couple ways. First, the act of eating, by itself, can release pent-up stress energy. Are you one of those people who like to eat crunchy foods when stressed? Turns out the physical act of chewing can help release stress energy. In addition, the act of eating a lot of food—of overeating or binge eating—actually forces the body to relax. Why? Well, stress and digestion are incompatible. When you are stressed, your body is not able to effectively digest food. So if you put enough food into the system, your body will say, "Hey, we need to deal with this now." It will force itself into relaxation chemistry in order to be able to begin digesting the heavy load.

So yeah, stress eating works. That's why we do it. Well, it kind of works. Eating can help relieve the stress we are feeling in the moment, but it doesn't affect whatever gave rise to the stress in the first place.

Engaging in stress eating once in a while is OK. However, when stress eating becomes a regular part of the everyday routine, our well-being can suffer. So let's look at ways to better manage our stress.

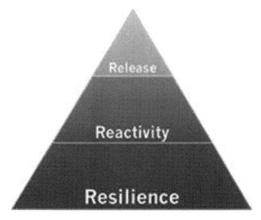

The Stress-Management Pyramid

In chapter three I introduced the stress-management pyramid. Here we'll explore each layer in detail so that you can

- build stress *resilience* to so that you reduce the frequency and impact of stress on your system,
- change how you *react* to situations so that you get triggered into stress less often, and
- create a larger menu of tools to *release* stress when it does occur.

RESILIENCE

Resilience is at the base of the stress-management pyramid because it is the foundation for your stress-management strategy. The more resilient to stress you can become, the less you need to worry about reactivity and release.

Resilience means cultivating a frame of mind and body that is resistant to stress. In other words, the more resilient your body is, the less frequently it will go into a stress response, and when it does enter stress chemistry, the impact will not be as great. Here are some ways to build stress resilience.

- *Mind-Body Nutrition.* All the techniques you have been working on so far—slowing down, being attentive, and being aware of who you are when you sit down to eat—contribute to building stress resilience. In addition, proper nutrition creates stress resilience. If your body regularly receives the vitamins, minerals, cofactors, phytonutrients, and adaptogens that it needs, it will be more stress-resilient. If you don't know what these terms mean, don't worry. Basically, it means eating a variety of simple, whole, nutrient-rich foods. On the other hand, if you eat a lot of nutrient-poor foods—foods containing processed sugars, flours, chemicals, and preservatives—your body will not be able to handle stress as well.

- *Meditation.* Research on meditation has shown a variety of health benefits. A regular meditation practice can contribute greatly to improving your stress resilience. Meditation is not difficult, but it is a practice (just like slowing down when you eat and all the other practices we are learning). You need to be consistent with it in order to reap the benefits. There are many tools and resources available to help you get started, including meditation apps, audio downloads, YouTube videos, and more.

- *Movement* is also key to managing stress and building stress resilience. Not only can movement release stress energy trapped in your system; it can also help you sleep better. The key here is to engage in movement that you enjoy.

For some, this may involve intense exercise. For others, it may involve practices like yoga or tai chi. Movement could be walking, dancing, working around the house, or gardening. But watch out—you can increase your stress through over-exercising or through engaging in movement activities that you don't like. So experiment and find out what resonates with you. And create some variety!

- *Sleep quality.* Poor sleep is a stress on your system. Getting quality sleep is also key to creating stress resilience.

- Other practices that can build stress resilience include spending time in nature, engaging in play (whatever that means to you—it could be playing sports or games, playing with children, or playing with pets), exploring your creativity, and journaling—keeping a gratitude journal, for example.

REACTIVITY

Would you believe that most of your stress is self-chosen? In other words, in a given situation, you are choosing (either consciously or subconsciously) to react in a stressful way.

You can't control everything that happens to you, but you can control how you react.

What if you could choose to react differently, in a way that's not stressful? What if you could shift your mind-set so that you were much less likely to react in a stressful way?

Key to creating this mind-set shift is improving your ability to see situations in different ways—that is, increasing your *cognitive flexibility*. When you are able to quickly and easily consider multiple perspectives, you give yourself the gift of choice. You have options. You can choose the perspective that allows you to react in a way that is more empowering and less stressful. Cognitive flexibility is a skill you can build using this simple exercise:

EXERCISE: COGNITIVE FLEXIBILITY
For a given situation, think of two or three plausible, positive alternative perspectives and associated reactions.

Example Situation: A driver cuts me off in traffic.

Perspective 1 (stressful): "That person obviously thinks he is more important than me. I'll honk the horn, tailgate him, and try to pull alongside him to give him a piece of my mind."

Perspective 2: "I wonder what that person is thinking about that makes him not able to pay attention to where he's going. I bet it's pretty important to him. I'm just glad I'm an alert, responsible driver and that I don't have his challenges."

Perspective 3: "I wonder what kind of emergency that driver might be rushing to. I'm glad all is well with me."

Perspective 4: "I'm so glad I'm not the kind of person who feels she needs to hurry all the time. Thank goodness my life isn't like that."

Example Situation: My boss walked right by me without acknowledging my presence.

Perspective 1 (stressful): "She must not value me as an employee. Am I really cut out for this job?"

Perspective 2: "She's really focused on something. Glad I didn't interrupt her concentration."

Perspective 3: "She looks to be in a hurry. I wonder if she's late for a meeting."

Once you start practicing cognitive flexibility, you begin seeing a whole host of alternative perspectives, ones that don't involve you at all. When the perspective doesn't involve you, you are released from the need to react.

I encourage you to practice cognitive flexibility over the next few days. Make it a game. How many alternative interpretations can you come up with for the situations you observe? Go ahead and have some fun with it. Maybe even go into the crazy, implausible realm. Why not? You're just practicing.

Release

No matter what, stress is going to happen. You can't avoid it completely. After all, that's why humans have a stress response. But when you notice you're feeling stressed, you can draw from a number of simple, effective techniques to move out of a stress response and into relaxation quite quickly.

- *Deep breathing.* The breath is an amazing tool. We don't usually give breathing much thought. It happens automatically. But the breath is tied to stress and relaxation in the following way. When we are stressed, our breath becomes shallow and rapid. When we are relaxed, our breath is slower and deeper. So to move us into relaxation, we just need to breathe slowly and deeply. The five-five-seven breathing technique, introduced earlier, is perfect for doing just that.

  Now, if you are really stressed, you may find it difficult to breathe deeply. That's because your stress response is wanting you to breathe rapidly and shallowly. If that happens, try starting your five-five-seven breathing with a quick count and then gradually slowing the count down. This will help you ease into relaxation.

- *Focus on relaxing thoughts.* Another technique to help you relax is to call up and focus on thoughts that relax you. This may be as simple as thinking about someone or something you love or something you are grateful for. Thoughts of love and gratitude can move you into relaxation. This is why we incorporated thoughts of gratitude into your practice from the previous chapter.

- *Visit your sanctuary.* Is there a place (real or imaginary) that evokes relaxation for you? Maybe it's a beach hut on a private island, a cabin in the woods, or the top of a mountain. Visualize this place in your mind, and visit it whenever you want to relax. While you are there, engage your senses—sight, sound, smell, and touch—to really ground yourself in this place. This is your happy place, your sanctuary, and it is available to you at any time.

- *Emotional freedom technique (EFT).* EFT, also known as tapping, was very instrumental to my binge-eating recovery and has become an important tool in my toolbox. Unfortunately, teaching EFT is beyond the scope of this book. If you are interested in learning more about EFT, you can find lots of resources online. I also offer EFT workshops (contact me if interested in exploring how to use EFT to transform your relationship with food).

Now you have a number of tools to help you build stress resilience, change your reactivity, and release stress. As you begin to practice some of these, observe how your desire to turn to food to manage stress changes.

Of course, stress isn't the only emotion that contributes to overeating. There are a number of other feelings that we don't like to experience, so we turn to food for relief. Let's look at what we can do about those.

Emotional overeating

If we are getting adequate sleep and nutrition, we aren't acting out of deprivation, and we aren't stressed, but we're still overeating, what do we do? To start, we need to recognize that overeating does not occur in a vacuum. There is some trigger or underlying cause. Everything we do is for some positive intention. So how is emotional overeating serving you? Discovering the underlying positive intention behind your emotional eating is an important first step in shifting that behavior.

Let's start to view emotional-eating instances as opportunities to learn about what needs to be addressed. Allow yourself to continue to use emotional eating as your go-to coping mechanism until you are in a position to try other strategies. But try to become more observant and curious, rather than judgmental. That's how we learn—through curiosity, not judgment.

Many people use emotional eating to cope with feelings they don't want to feel or to satisfy unmet needs. The habit of reaching for food in this way can be so automatic that you don't even give yourself a chance to slow down and identify what your trigger is. Be patient with yourself. Part of you is wanting to bring attention to this situation. Allow it to come forward.

There are two key questions that you can ask yourself to help you discover what is triggering you and what you can do about it.

The first is, "What am I feeling now?"

Ask yourself this question as you are reaching for food. Are you physically hungry? Are you experiencing the signs of physical hunger (such as an empty, growling stomach)? If so, then choose something to eat (the next chapter addresses what you should choose).

If you aren't physically hungry, is there a particular emotion that you are experiencing? Here are some you might be feeling:

Fearful, anxious, edgy, frightened, nervous, scared, wary, worried, angry, irritated, outraged, resentful, sad, dejected, depressed, empty, gloomy, grief, hopeless, lonely, bored, apathetic, indifferent, restless, disgusted, appalled, contempt, disdain, indignant, repulsed, revolted, shocked, startled, dumbfounded, astonished, joyful, amused, happy.

If none of these seems quite right, try *uncomfortable* to see if that resonates.

It might be helpful to explore what you are feeling in your body. Emotional energy creates certain body sensations. For example, sadness may create a tight, heavy feeling in the chest. Anger may manifest as tension in the body. Other feelings can be reflected by certain sensations in the abdomen. By exploring how the emotional energy manifests in your body, you are drawing attention to it and acknowledging it, which can help you identify it and even release it!

Keep in mind that whatever you are feeling is true and valid for you. Your feelings do not need to be justified or judged. There's no "I shouldn't feel this way."

The the reality is: you do! Why argue with reality? Acknowledge what you are feeling, own it, and then take the next step.

It's OK if you're unsure exactly how to label what it is that you are feeling. The very act of asking the question is progress. You are slowing down to ask and to listen. Answers will come in time.

The next question to ask is, "What do I need now?" Here are some options to consider:

DISTRACTION
Sometimes we can distract ourselves long enough to allow the uncomfortable feeling to dissipate on its own. However, if there is an underlying issue that will continue to trigger that feeling, that issue will remain.

Ways to distract: change your environment, watch something funny, go to a store or out with a friend, play with a pet, listen to music, read a book, do a puzzle, work on a craft, or color in a coloring book.

SUPPORT
Being able to talk about the feeling, rather than avoid it through food, can be quite effective. Most people do not reach out for support because they are afraid of being a burden. Think about how you feel when you get to help

someone. By reaching out for support, you are giving someone else the opportunity to make herself feel better by providing you with the support you are looking for.

You could call, text, e-mail, or message a friend or family member. You could chat online or connect with someone via social media, or you could even talk to a coach, counselor, therapist, or spiritual advisor. The important thing is to create that connection along which energy can flow.

SELF-CARE

Sometimes what is needed is a little self-care. Women especially are so used to putting everyone and everything else first that they don't take time for themselves—or they feel guilty doing so. Could the need for self-care be manifesting through overeating? Absolutely.

Self-care can consist of taking a nap, taking a relaxing bath, going for a walk outside, meditating, giving yourself the gift of some alone time, or unplugging from electronics.

PROCESS THE FEELING

Often emotional eating is used to distract or numb us from feeling an uncomfortable feeling. So how do we remove the need to emotionally eat? We allow ourselves to process the feeling. Here are some ways to do so.

- *Feel the feeling,* also known as "getting comfortable with being uncomfortable." Breathe deeply and sit with it. Notice how it feels in your body. Where does it show up? In the chest? Stomach? Head? Neck? What's going on physically? As you exhale, picture healing breath flowing to the area of sensation. Perhaps say to yourself something like, "In this moment, I am safe."

- *Keep a journal.* Journaling is a great tool for processing feelings. I view journaling as the "fiber for your emotions" because it helps move emotions through your body, just like fiber helps food move through your digestive tract. Notice "emotion" has the word "motion" in it. I like to think of emotions as energy in motion—e-motion. If we don't allow the energy to move, and if we don't allow ourselves to feel it, then the energy gets stuck. We become emotionally constipated. Journaling is one way to help move the energy. When you journal an emotion, write whatever comes to mind. No editing, no censoring.

- *Write a letter.* If your feeling is tied to a person, you could write that person a letter. It might be helpful to decide, in advance, that you are going to write a letter that you never intend to send. In fact, when you finish writing the letter, you can ceremonially destroy it in whatever way feels right—shred it, flush it, or burn it. If your feeling is not associated with a specific person, you can always write a letter to yourself—perhaps to that part of yourself that is responsible for triggering the feeling.

- *Noticing.* This is a mindfulness practice that encourages you to detach from the feeling and just observe it. Here's the idea. When you feel a triggering thought or emotion, picture it as a puffy cloud in the sky that you are watching from a safe distance, maybe you're inside your house watching it through a window. You acknowledge its existence. Maybe you even talk to it—gently. "Ah, there you are again." But you remain a detached observer. Importantly, you don't go into the thought. You don't become attached to it, and you don't engage it or pursue it. And when the breeze blows that cloud away, you just let it go.
- *Emotional freedom technique* (EFT) is a great tool for moving emotional energy—and lots of other things too! If you know it, use it! If you don't, I invite you to explore it.
- Finally, you can talk to a healer, coach, counselor, or other professional who can help you process the emotion.

Through these techniques, what we're aiming to do is to allow the emotion—the energy—to move through the body, like a wave, instead of trying to dam it up. Conversation, journaling, observing with detachment, and EFT are all tools to encourage the energy to move. Physical activity (like yoga, tai chi, chi gong, and others) can also help release trapped emotions.

Concluding thoughts

Transforming emotional eating behavior is a complex and personal process. If it were that simple, there wouldn't be so many books about it, right? My goal here has been to help you build a solid foundation from which to explore deeper, if you need to. Through your work on the activities in this chapter, it is my hope that you will become more comfortable with where you are at, create increased awareness around how you use food emotionally, and acquire some new tools to help you work with your emotions. However, often what is required is deeper healing, which can be most effectively done in the context of private work with a coach, counselor, or other healer.

For example, you may become more aware of what your emotional triggers are, and you may become better prepared to react to them in a nonfood fashion. What you might want to explore next is a deeper question: why do those emotional triggers arise for me? Why do I keep feeling anger, anxiety, or sadness? What can I do to heal whatever is giving rise to these feelings? If that's a journey you are looking to go on, I invite you to connect with me.

Takeaways

Here are the key takeaways from this chapter:

- Eating for reasons other than hunger is natural.
- However, turning to food to manage your emotions can become an overused strategy, which can then detract from your health and well-being.
- The goal isn't to eliminate emotional eating entirely but to reduce one's dependence on it by providing additional tools for managing the uncomfortable emotions.
- We explored overeating as
  - a result of sleep or nutrient deficiency,
  - a reaction to deprivation,
  - a strategy for managing stress, and
  - a strategy for avoiding uncomfortable feelings.

Your activities in this chapter are designed to help you build awareness around what feelings trigger emotional eating for you and what you can do to manage those feelings without turning to food.

Activities

There are five activities designed to help you explore your relationship with emotional eating, increase awareness and mindfulness, and create some emotional resilience. Here is how I suggest you work through them.

- Start with the first journaling activity. As with all journaling activities, this may be one that you complete in one sitting or in multiple sittings. You may want to come back and add to it as more insights arise.
- Once you have made progress with the first activity, proceed to the second. I suggest you pick a couple of days (or more) where you make this your focus.
- When you feel you have a good handle on the second, add the third to the mix. Now you will be essentially working on the second and third at the same time. Again, focus on this for a couple of days or more—whatever time frame feels right for you.
- Now that you are familiar with what you have been feeling and when, you can begin working on the fourth exercise. My recommendation would be to try this exercise once a day, while you continue to practice activities two and three.
- Once you have explored activities one through four, you can proceed to the fifth.

1. YOUR RELATIONSHIP WITH EMOTIONAL EATING

In your journal, write about your relationship with emotional eating. What do you remember about how the connection between food and emotion has shown up in your life? How has emotional eating served you? Would you like to change your relationship with emotional eating?

If you like, you can write this as a letter to yourself. For example: "Dear Dawn, I don't know if you realized this, but you are an emotional eater—and that's OK. I notice it started back when _____ because you needed _____."

2. WHAT ARE YOU FEELING?

The goal of this activity is to cultivate a closer connection to your body and to increase your presence and awareness by checking in regularly to see what you are feeling.

What I'd like you to do is pause several times during your day (you may want to set up a reminder on your phone) and check in by asking, "What am I feeling now?"

Ask the question from a place of curiosity. Acknowledge that whatever you are feeling right now is valid and true. Take care you don't fall into judgmental thoughts like, "I shouldn't be feeling this way," or "I wish I were feeling…" The reality is you are feeling whatever you are feeling. Don't argue with reality!

What we're trying to do here is raise awareness around and validate your range of feelings. We aren't trying to ask why you are feeling a certain way. We aren't trying to justify, and we aren't trying to change.

3. WHAT ARE YOU FEELING BEFORE YOU EAT?

While the previous activity asked you to check in at various times during the day to observe what you are feeling, this activity focuses specifically on becoming aware of what you are feeling before you eat. It also has the benefit of creating an important pause before you begin eating— a pause that creates the opportunity for you to be more mindful about your choices.

Here's what I'd like you to do. Before you begin eating a meal or a snack, pause to ask yourself, "What am I feeling? Am I feeling hunger? If so, how strong is it? Am I feeling something else?"

After you explore these questions, you have a choice. You may choose to eat, whether to satisfy true hunger or for emotional reasons. Or you may choose to ask, "What do I need now?"

Then experiment with a nonfood activity to address that need.

Note: even if you choose to eat when you aren't hungry, you are still making that choice from a place of mindfulness, rather than from a place of uncontrollable habit.

4. FEEL YOUR FEELINGS

One way to loosen your dependence on emotional eating is to become more comfortable with those feelings that you've been using food to avoid. Or as I like to say, become more comfortable with being uncomfortable. In this activity, you'll practice sitting with your uncomfortable feelings. Think of this as an exercise that will be strengthening your emotional-resilience muscle.

Pick a particular feeling you want to work on—one that has been a challenge for you. Maybe it's one you identified when you explored your relationship with emotional eating in the first activity. Find a safe, quiet place where you can explore comfortably. Use your imagination to call up that feeling. Maybe you remember a past situation where it came up, or you imagine a situation where it might come up. Call up the feeling, and see if you can amplify it. Dial it up as high as you can.

As you are feeling this feeling, breathe deeply, and explore with curiosity:

- "Where do I feel this in my body?"
- "What is uncomfortable about this feeling?"

- "Knowing that I am safe in this moment, and knowing that this feeling will pass, am I OK to tolerate this feeling a little longer?"
- "Next time I am feeling like this, what might I be able to do to move this feeling through my body?"

5. WHAT HAVE YOU LEARNED?

In your journal, reflect on what you learned in this chapter. What did you learn about yourself and who you would like to be?

Eight

JUST TELL ME WHAT TO EAT!

I remember one time during my binge-eating days, I stopped in a Walmart. As I was walking through the store, I came across a display of Pepperidge Farm cookies—Limited Edition Seasonal Flavors!

My mind went into that place of, "I just have to have them. I need to experience them. If I don't have them now, I'll never have the chance again, and I'll miss out."

And so they ended up in the cart.

I opened them up as soon as I got into the car, thinking, "I'll just have one or two and bring the rest home to share." Well, I ended up eating almost all of them. Then I had to throw the rest away because I couldn't bring home an almost empty package of cookies!

Incidents like these reveal that I was making food choices based on scarcity, deprivation, and even fear. Or when I wasn't binging, I was choosing foods based on what would fit within the confines of whatever diet program I was following.

Now I engage with food quite differently. I make choices based on how my body will feel. I don't really think about my choices too much. When I'm feeling hungry, I just do a quick check-in to feel into what my body needs and wants, to see what would make it feel good—not just in the immediate moment but over time. And it almost always gives me a clear answer. That's my intuitive-eating muscle doing its work.

F inally, we are going to address the *what* of eating. If I had a dollar for every time someone said, "Just tell me what to eat," let's just say I'd be quite well off by now. And perhaps you, dear reader, have grown frustrated because you want to know this too. So why have I left this for last?

Well, I hope by now you've come to appreciate that there is much more to a healthy relationship with food than just what you choose to eat on a regular basis. Unfortunately, most diet programs focus primarily on the "what" of eating. I mean, you can get diet meals shipped right to your door! Given that diets fail over 95 percent of the time, clearly there is something missing from that approach.

That's why we addressed the other dimensions of your relationship with food first—the how, when, where, who, and why. In fact, understanding and appreciating those other dimensions is key to what we are going to focus on here: how to discover what to eat for your unique body and how to strengthen your intuitive-eating muscle so that making food choices becomes no big deal.

Would you be surprised to learn that there's no simple answer to the question, "What should I eat?" Not only is every body unique, but in order to cultivate a sustainable nourishing eating style, it's important to consider:

- *Personal preferences.* What foods do you enjoy?
- *Lifestyle.* How and when do you create time for shopping and meal prep? Does it make sense for you to cook meals ahead of time?

- *Activity level.* How do you need to adapt your food choices to accommodate more and less active days?
- *How your body reacts to different foods.* Are there certain foods that you might be sensitive to?

Don't worry, though. I'm going to lead you through a process that will allow you to tune in on your own personal eating style. Here's how we're going to proceed.

We'll begin by introducing four guidelines to help you make food choices. Then we'll look at how you can put these guidelines into practice. Along the way, we'll touch upon fun things like pleasure, food morality, supplementation, food sensitivities, and more.

Are you ready? Let's dive in!

Guidelines for making food choices

Ultimately, the goal is to be able to choose the best foods for our bodies automatically and intuitively. In reality, though, we've been inundated with so many rules and bits of information about food and diets from "experts" and the media that our heads are swimming. Part of your journey to a peaceful relationship with food is to let go of these external influences. Once you let go, you create room for the natural intuitive eater in you to reawaken.

We began the process of letting go right away, in chapter two, and have continued that process throughout. And we have been slowly awakening your intuitive eater through the practices that we have been introducing. Here we introduce four guidelines that will help you tap into your body's intuition and strengthen your intuitive muscle even more. So without further ado, let's introduce the first guideline.

GUIDELINE 1: CHOOSE EMPOWERING FOODS THAT MAKE YOU FEEL YOUR BEST

We all want to feel good, right? Well, would it surprise you to learn that how we feel is hugely affected by what we eat? I didn't' think so.

But we don't often make that connection. We get so busy running here and there, involved in our work and our day-to-day things, that we don't really pay attention to our bodies' signals. Or when we do notice something awry, we ingest something else (fast food, an energy drink, a painkiller, a heartburn remedy, and so on) to try to alleviate the symptom without thinking about how that symptom came about.

What we eat affects our energy, sleep, mood, hunger, cravings, and physical comfort. Our food choices can cause digestive distress, aches and pains in the joints, brain fog, and low energy. Or our food choices can give us steady energy, keep us alert and focused, promote restful sleep, and keep us in a good mood.

Which would you prefer?

I thought so.

But this guideline begs the question: What are empowering foods, and what does "best" mean?

Empowering foods are ones that enable you to have good energy, restful sleep, a steady mood, manageable hunger and cravings, and physical comfort. These are your body's feedback signals. These are your signposts. The work from the previous chapters has set you up so you are now better prepared to notice and pay attention to these signals.

Which specific foods create this "best" feeling will vary from one person to the next. We'll explore this in more detail later. For now let's start with this generalization:

The foods that tend to have an empowering effect are nutrient-dense, high-quality, whole (single-ingredient) foods with minimal processing.

Now consider a corollary to our first guideline.

Corollary: Minimize disempowering foods that make you feel *blech*

Notice this doesn't say "never eat." But why would you want to regularly eat foods that drain your energy, make you feel lethargic, put you in a bad mood, give you heartburn or indigestion, or cause you to feel bloated or achy? That's no fun.

Again, which foods make you feel *blech* will vary from individual to individual. Often, disempowering foods are ones that are highly processed, with many ingredients, some of which you may not be able to pronounce. These foods may contain various forms of sugar (natural or artificial), white flour, processed, low-quality fats, preservatives, and other chemicals.

Now remember, there are no good foods or bad foods. There's just food. We aren't trying to label foods as good or bad here. Some we like, and some we don't. Some make us feel good, and some don't. Some empower us, and some don't. We're trying to bring awareness to the idea that different foods affect us in different ways. And we want to choose what makes us feel good most of the time.

What you'll notice is that as you incorporate more of the foods that make you feel good, you'll naturally crowd out the ones that don't. It's not that you will be depriving yourself of those foods. They just won't have the same appeal.

GUIDELINE 2: CHOOSE THE HIGHEST QUALITY YOU CAN IN THE SITUATION YOU ARE IN

This second guideline is about refining your food choices a little bit and, at the same time, creating a feeling of flexibility. The idea is that when you are selecting your foods, you want to choose the highest quality within your means, given the situation.

For example, when choosing produce, try to select fresh (or freshly frozen), organic foods that are locally grown and harvested and minimally processed. For animal products, try to choose products from naturally fed and humanely raised animals, free of growth hormone and antibiotics. For fish products, look for fish caught in the wild and low in heavy metals like mercury. There are different quality options for all food types, including oils, nuts, seeds, everything!

Often when I talk about food quality, I hear objections like, "It costs too much money," "High-quality foods are too hard to find," or "They are too inconvenient." And of course, there is some truth to that.

But often underlying these objections, there's a little bit of "I'm not worth it. I'm not worth the extra money or the extra time," or "I don't deserve to have high-quality things." If that resonates with you at all, then my question for you is this: what do you need to do to be worth it or to be deserving? What makes other people deserving but not you?

Of course, you are as worthy and deserving as anyone. Giving yourself permission to choose high-quality foods for yourself (and your family) can help you let go of some of the attachments you have to thoughts of being unworthy or undeserving. When you let those thoughts go, your self-esteem and confidence naturally rise. Because you are worth it. You do deserve it. So go for it!

What I love about this guideline is its flexibility. Let's face it. Sometimes we find ourselves in situations where our favorite foods, the high-quality ones that make us feel great, just aren't available. For example, we may be traveling, at a party, or at a restaurant. In these situations, you still get to make the choice that is going to make you feel your best, whatever that means to you in the situation. You get to make a choice free of guilt or shame or the feeling of "rule violation." Just remember who you are as you are enjoying these foods—someone who is relaxed, who knows her body will efficiently extract the nutrition it needs, and who will feel nourished nonetheless.

Let's introduce our third guideline. I think you'll really like this one. Before I introduce it, I want to ask you this: how much to you enjoy what you eat? Are you choosing foods that give you pleasure?

When I was dieting, my "staple" meal was grilled chicken, steamed broccoli, and plain brown rice. And then there were the diet foods—fat-free this, cardboard that. Not much pleasure there at all. No wonder when I came across food that tasted really good I ended up over-eating. I was pleasure deprived.

You see, we are wired to seek pleasure and avoid pain. To seek the pleasure of food and avoid the pain of hunger. And thus, our third guideline now follows.

GUIDELINE 3: SEEK PLEASURE AND SATISFACTION

Why do we need this guideline? It helps us from feeling deprived. Especially for those who may still be in the process of letting go of diet culture, it can be extremely liberating to acknowledge that pleasure and satisfaction are important to our well-being. The guideline, in some sense, gives us permission to do something that is natural to us but that we may have denied ourselves for a long time.

The importance of pleasure from eating is backed up by research. Pleasure increases metabolic efficiency, meaning pleasure increases your ability to absorb and as-similate the nutrients in your food so that your body gets what it needs. And when your body gets what it needs, it rewards you with feelings of fullness and satisfaction and with good energy, mood, sleep, and more.

For example, in one study, women were fed a regular meal one day and then the same meal in blended form (the food was placed in a blender and processed until smooth) a different day. Both times, the researchers measured the absorption of iron and found that when the meal was blended, iron absorption decreased by up to 70 percent. It was suggested that this decrease could be attributed to a lack of pleasure—subjects didn't like the blended version of the meal.

If we look at what happens chemically when we experience pleasure, it turns out that the same chemical (cholecystokinin, CCK) responsible for stimulating the sensation of pleasure in the brain also aids digestion by stimulating the small intestine, pancreas, gallbladder, and stomach and shuts down appetite. In other words, the same chemical that helps us metabolize our meal is also involved in telling us when we've had enough, and it makes us feel good about the experience.

Finally, pleasure is incompatible with stress. When you are under stress, you can't experience pleasure. This is another reason why it's important to be a relaxed eater.

In sum, if you deny yourself the pleasure of food, through low-calorie eating, consuming bland diet foods, or a fun-free diet, your appetite won't be satisfied. So go ahead—add a bit of butter, salt, sugar, and spice to make your food taste nice. Your brain and body will thank you.

Now let's now turn to our fourth and final guideline.

GUIDELINE 4: ASK YOUR BODY WHAT IT WANTS

When you are feeling hungry and deciding what to eat, why not ask your body? That's where the hunger is coming from, after all.

What do I mean by asking your body?

What I encourage clients to do is start by taking a deep breath or two to help you relax and open up to hearing your body. Then picture different food options while holding a question in your mind like, "Is this what will satisfy my body?" or "Is this what my body is wanting right now?" What you're looking for is a feeling of "Yes, that will do" or "No, that's not it." We are looking for that answer to come from the body, not from the mind.

This may sound a little woo-woo, but it works—if you've cultivated that connection with your body that this book is guiding you to do and if you take the time to relax and listen.

Asking your body in this way is a practice. As with most practices you've learned in this book, at first this one may feel a little forced, and you may not receive a response from your body. The body may not be used to being considered in this way. It may be used to being ignored. So it may take some time for the body to respond. But it will. In fact, over time, this process can become so automatic that you are able to just look at or picture a food and instantly receive feedback from your body about how that food will work out for you.

And you know what? If nothing appeals, then your body probably isn't really hungry. You're most likely experiencing a different kind of "hunger"—perhaps an emotional one. In that case, begin exploring nonfood choices and see what lands for you.

To summarize, the four guidelines are the following:

1. Choose empowering foods that make you feel best.
2. Choose the highest quality you can in the situation you're in.
3. Seek out pleasure and satisfaction.
4. Ask your body what it wants.

Discover your own eating style

Let's look at how you can apply these guidelines to create an eating style that's just right for you. The process is actually quite simple. Before we get into the details, I want to emphasize that what we are doing here is creating a flexible way of eating that is adaptable based on the body's needs. Some days the body will need more food;

other days it will need less food. We are putting together all that we know about the how, when, where, who, and why to help us determine the what.

The goal is not to create a specific meal plan with recipes and ingredients. Nor are we looking to count or measure anything. And we're definitely not creating a set of unbreakable rules. Instead, we are looking to use our bodies' feedback systems to adjust and eat in a way that makes us feel good.

YOUR BODY'S FEEDBACK SYSTEM

These are the five main signals we'll be paying attention to: hunger, energy, cravings, mood, and sleep. You should also attend to other symptoms that might arise, such as bloating, indigestion, irregular bowel movements, aches and pains in the joints, brain fog, and so on, as these could be the result of something you ate (we'll return to discuss these later).

To discover your own eating style, we'll be uncovering your empowering foods and exploring how to best combine them.

WHAT ARE YOUR EMPOWERING FOODS?

Your empowering foods are the ones that make you feel your best. These are the foods that you want to be eating regularly. But which ones are they?

To begin answering this question, I'd like you to get out a piece of paper and make two columns: "Foods that give me energy" and "Foods that take energy away."

Now begin filling in those columns. It's OK if you can't think of any or if you are unsure. Do the best you can at this stage. You can continue adding to the list over time.

Now take a look at what you've come up with. Are there any generalizations you can draw about the foods in the two columns? Any characteristics they share? What other foods might share these characteristics? The answer to the latter can help you pinpoint some foods you might want to experiment with.

You can also make analogous lists that focus how food affects your hunger and cravings, mood, satisfaction, pleasure, and even sleep. Which foods keep you fuller longer? Which ones might lead to increased cravings or mood swings? This exploration is all about increasing your knowledge around how different foods affect you and strengthening your mind-body connection.

Please understand we aren't creating a list of good foods and bad foods. We are just acknowledging that food affects us in certain ways and bringing awareness to which foods affect you in which way. Your list is unique to you. While my list may overlap somewhat with yours, there will be differences.

What you're aiming to do is recognize which foods make you feel your best, give you the best energy, and so on, and which foods make you not feel so good. And not just in the short term, but over time. So when you are considering how you are affected by a food, try to think longer term—maybe hours later or even the next day.

For example, if you feel an energy dip, think about the last time you ate and what you ate. How might that have contributed to your dip? Maybe it's time to just refuel again, or maybe you ate something that drained your energy. Or maybe you did something else that drained your energy. Being aware of your body allows you to ask these questions.

I like to call the foods that end up in the left column the "eat regularly" foods and the ones in the right column the "eat occasionally (or rarely)" foods.

Knowledge is power. By going through this kind of activity, by becoming more aware of which foods affect you and how, you get to make conscious, informed food choices. When you understand how food makes you feel, not just in the moment but over a longer period of time, and when you focus on how you want to feel over a longer period of time, you will naturally gravitate toward choosing those foods that make you feel best most of the time. And those tend to be the choices that are healthiest for your unique body. Makes sense, right?

Of course, the foods in the right column are still available to you. You may find you have them occasionally or rarely—whatever feels right for you. But when you have them, you choose them with the knowledge that your body will react in a certain way, and you are OK with that. You have the power to choose.

I encourage you to also create a list of foods that give you pleasure and satisfaction. Experiencing pleasure from food is an important part of a healthy relationship with food. As you create this list, notice which of your pleasure foods show up on your "eat regularly" lists versus which ones show up on your "have occasionally" lists. Also notice whether you avoided adding certain foods to your pleasure list because part of you still feels they are "triggers" or "bad" or you think, "I can never have that in the house." Those are dieter's thoughts. As long as you hold on to those thoughts, those foods will have control over you. Add those foods to your list, and put asterisks next to them, as you have some work to do around them. Don't worry. I have an activity for you to work on that.

FOOD COMBINING

In addition to knowing how various individual foods affect your body, how foods are combined has a dramatic impact as well. For example, you may find that when a food that by itself robs you of energy is combined with other foods, the effect is lessened, perhaps even to the extent that there is no effect at all.

I encourage you to explore how different food combinations affect your body. Specifically, by food combinations, I'm referring to the combination of food types: proteins, carbohydrates, and fats. What you are trying to do, again, is discover the combination (or combinations) that works well for you. I call your favored food combination your *Magic Plate*. This is the combination that gives you steady energy, a healthy appetite with few cravings, good sleep, and a good mood.

Here's how you can discover your Magic Plate.

1. START WITH A GENERIC MAGIC PLATE

I recommend you begin by aiming to have your meals composed of about half (by volume) nonstarchy vegetables, one-quarter protein, one-quarter healthy carbs, plus some healthy fat mixed in. I'm not asking you to measure your food. What I'm suggesting is that if you were to lay your meal out on a plate, it might look like the picture you see below. In other words, when you look at the volume of food on your plate, about half of it would be composed of nonstarchy vegetables and the like. The healthy carb component could be a starchy vegetable like potato or corn, a grain (rice, quinoa, and so on), fruit, or even bread. A healthy fat might be olive oil, coconut oil, nuts, nut butter, butter, or ghee.

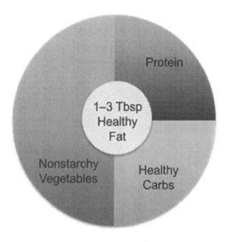

If you already have an intuition about what your Magic Plate looks like, feel free to start with that.

Of course, you'll be

- asking your body what it wants,
- choosing your "regular" foods (most of the time),
- choosing the highest quality versions of those that you can, and

- remembering to include a little something that will make the meal pleasurable.

And you'll be eating slowly, with attentiveness, while sitting down and being a relaxed, grateful eater. You'll eat when you are hungry, to the point of satisfaction.

2. MAKE ADJUSTMENTS

The Magic Plate is a starting guideline. It's up to you to pay attention to how that plate, as an eating style, works for you. You see, the same Magic Plate isn't going to work for everybody. Some people need more carbs, and some need less. Some people need more fat, and some need less. Some people enjoy lots of veggies, and others don't.

How do you know if the Magic Plate is working for you? You monitor your body's feedback system: hunger, energy, cravings, mood, and sleep. If these indicators all feel good to you, then there's no need to make any changes. Just continue to eat in this style most of the time. But if something feels out of alignment, if you notice over a period of a few days that one of these indicators is off, then you can experiment with making adjustments. Try the following tweaks, in the order given.

1. Add more protein, fiber (through vegetables), and water.
2. Add more fat.

3. Add more healthy carbs.
4. Add a snack.

Scenario: You find yourself feeling hungry within two hours of having breakfast.

Should you make an adjustment to your breakfast Magic Plate? Well, it depends on how this feels for you. Are you OK with experiencing hunger at this point (and responding to it by eating something)? Or is it difficult given your lifestyle to have something to eat at this time? Depending on how you answer, you may or may not want to adjust your breakfast. If you choose to do so, try the options given, starting at the top of the list. Run your experiment for a few days and see what happens.

Notice how this works. It starts with an observation that something isn't quite working for you. So you make an adjustment, and test it out. When you experiment, test your adjustment for at least a few days, or perhaps even a week. If the adjustment helps, then that becomes your new Magic Plate.

You may actually end up having different Magic Plates for different meals. For example, in my case, my breakfast Magic Plate is typically higher in protein and lower in veggies and carbs than my other meals. My breakfast typically consists of a protein shake, with fat, carbs, and veggies mixed in. This works great for me. It holds me all the way through lunch on most days. I have noticed that if I eat oatmeal for breakfast, I get hungry a lot sooner. Well, oatmeal is mainly carbs. So I've learned to add some protein and fat to it (chocolate protein powder and almond butter, for example), which gives me much better sustained energy throughout the morning.

Give yourself permission to create different Magic Plates for different meals. Remember the guidelines. Ultimately, the goal is to feel good, honor your hunger and fullness, and make informed choices that are going to support you in having an amazing day and an amazing life.

Think of this process of creating your eating style as an experiment. You are the scientist making observations and collecting data. Be curious, and have fun.

One more thing. You may find your Magic Plate, whatever it ends up looking like, works for you for six months or a year. But your body is constantly changing, and your activity is changing; hence, your nutritional needs will change too. Remaining open and curious and flexible is important. Once you work this process for a while, it becomes second nature. You end up adjusting your eating without even thinking about it. That's the joy of being an intuitive eater.

On snacking

Notice that one of the adjustments is to add in snacks. Snacking is an area that is quite controversial in the nutritional world. All kinds of rules have been proposed—for example, "No snacks allowed," "You must have snacks between meals," or "No snacks allowed after seven at night." These are all rules—and you know what we think about rules, right?

I encourage you to think of snacking as a tool to help you honor your hunger. You may find that you need to snack regularly, or not at all, or only on some days.

You may also decide at times to practice "preemptive snacking." This is when you plan a snack in anticipation that events or your schedule will prevent you from having a proper meal when your body would normally want it.

What should you choose for a snack? Well, I like to think of a snack as a mini meal—a mini Magic Plate. In other words, you want to try to have a snack that includes a combination of protein, fat, and carbs.

Food sensitivities

Before we conclude this chapter, I'd like to briefly address food sensitivities. It's important to recognize that anybody can be sensitive to just about any food. I'm not talking about food allergies, but food sensitivities.

Common sensitivities include gluten, dairy, eggs, soy, citrus, and nightshades. Symptoms of food sensitivities run a wide gamut—indigestion, bloating, aches and pains in the joints, chronic congestion, brain fog, low energy, and more.

We are seeing a rise in food sensitivities in our society. Food sensitivities can come and go. They can be the result of inherent body characteristics (e.g., maybe the body doesn't produce a particular enzyme needed to digest a protein found in a particular food). Sensitivities can also result from damage to the digestive tract. A main source of digestive-tract damage is stress.

Continuing to eat foods to which your body is sensitive can lead to more serious conditions down the road. So it's important to identify any foods to which you might be sensitive. However, food sensitivities are difficult to detect through medical testing. The medical tests just aren't sensitive enough yet. They can tell you that you are sensitive to something (which usually indicates a high degree of sensitivity), but they can't tell you that you are not. But your body knows. Your body is the ultimate authority for whether you are sensitive to a food or not, independent of what any medical test might say!

One way to identify food sensitivities is to use a simple elimination-reintroduction protocol. This involves eliminating a test food group for a period of time and then reintroducing it and monitoring symptoms. If you think you have food sensitivities, I recommend you go through an elimination-reintroduction program to identify the foods to which you are sensitive before you begin experimenting with building your own eating style. My fourteen-day Mind-Body Reset coaching program includes an elimination-reintroduction protocol to help with this.

Summary

The biggest takeaway from this chapter is this:

Your body is the ultimate authority for any eating strategy you choose.

It's not what the experts say or what I say. It's what your body says. How do different foods and food combinations affect your hunger, energy, cravings, mood, and sleep? These are the signposts that can guide you in making the choices that are best for you.

I offered you four guidelines for choosing the foods that are best for you:

1. Choose empowering foods that make you feel your best.
2. Choose the highest quality you can in the situation you're in.
3. Seek out pleasure and satisfaction.
4. Ask your body what it wants.

By following these guidelines, you will learn which foods give you good energy, stable hunger, good sleep, and so on. As you become more attuned to how different foods affect your body, you will naturally gravitate toward those that make you feel your best over time. These will become your regular foods. However, you will still incorporate your infrequent foods for flexibility, pleasure, and satisfaction.

We then turned to the application of these guidelines to help you create an eating style just for you, by

1. identifying which foods work best for you and
2. discovering your Magic Plate.

Your activities for this chapter are designed to help you examine your current eating style and make any adjustments you think are necessary.

Remember as you are working through the activities to use all the skills and tools you have been learning—to relax and eat slowly, with attention, and to the point of satisfaction. It's these skills that will help you notice your body's feedback and use it to your advantage.

Now it's time to put this into action!

Activities

1. Explore which foods work best for you
Create lists of your *regular foods* and your *occasional foods*, using the process described in this chapter. Focus first on how foods affect you energetically. Then focus on hunger. Give yourself permission to build these lists over time.

2. What are your pleasure foods?
Create a list of your pleasure foods. Make sure you include any foods that you feel are "triggers" or "bad" or that you "could never have in the house," and put an asterisk next to them.

How do your pleasure foods relate to the lists you created in the previous exercise? Which pleasure foods are on the *regular* list and which are on the *occasional* list?

3. Practice pleasure from food!
Have at least one pleasure food this week. Is there one you haven't had in a long time, one that you've been avoiding

because it's been a "trouble" food for you in the past? Do you have any asterisked foods on your pleasure food list? If so, pick one of those. Create a plan for enjoying that food—mindfully, in the presence of others, if you can.

Journal what this experience was like. What thoughts came to mind before you had the food? Did you enjoy it as much as you thought you would, or perhaps even more? How did you feel afterward? How did your body react?

4. What is your Magic Plate?

Think about your regular eating patterns. What does your Magic Plate look like now? Do you have different Magic Plates for different meals? Do you feel your Magic Plates are working for you? Do you want to experiment with a different one? If so, use the process outlined in the chapter to play with your Magic Plate. I suggest you focus on one meal at a time, starting with your first meal of the day: breakfast.

5. What have you learned?

In your journal, write about what you learned in this chapter. What did you learn about yourself and who you would like to be?

Nine

NOW WHAT?

I can't remember the last time I went into a cupcake store. Not because I restrict myself, but because I have realized that cupcakes don't actually taste that good to me, at least not anymore. Even more importantly, they don't make me feel so good in my body.

I eat when I'm hungry, and most of the time, I stop when I'm full. Sometimes that means I have lunch at 11:15 a.m., sometimes at 1:30 p.m. In fact, I don't always differentiate between a meal and a snack. I check in with my body, and it gives me an idea of how much food it is wanting.

I don't think of foods as good or bad, or healthy or unhealthy. I know there are certain foods that I do

*not like. Some of them would be considered "healthy"
by the general population—and others not.*

*Most significantly, food decisions are not stressful,
guilt-ridden experiences like they used to be. Food
just doesn't hold the charge that it used to. Don't get
me wrong: I still love to eat. But food is no longer a
daily struggle for me.*

*Words feel inadequate for conveying how amazing
it feels to be free.*

*People often ask me how long it took for me to get
where I am, to become the intuitive eater that I am
today. I think they ask because they want to know
who long it might take them. But I don't know how
to answer that question. It's not like I woke up one day
and said, "Yes, I've arrived!" The change happened
little by little. And I had a lot of help along the way.*

*I was born an intuitive eater. It's always been inside
me. It went dormant for a while, but now, thankfully, it is awake again.*

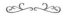

And so we have reached the end of the book but not
the end of the journey. I encourage you to continue

the practices you have learned here. The path to peace with food happens in small, gradual steps. It requires patience, compassion, and forgiveness. And the rewards are tremendous.

What do I hope you have taken away from this book? A conviction to never diet again. Awareness that there is a lot more to a healthy relationship with food than just what you eat. Determination to continue on the path of peace, despite the influence of the surrounding diet culture. And perhaps acknowledgment that the path is not one that you need to journey alone.

If you would like to be supported as you continue your journey, I encourage you to reach out to me. I would love to share a conversation with you that could help you on your journey.

Recommended Reading

Bacon, Linda. 2008. *Health at Every Size: The Surprising Truth about Your Weight.* Dallas, TX: BenBella Books.

Bacon, Linda, and Lucy Aphramor. 2011. "Weight Science: Evaluating the Evidence for a Paradigm Shift." *Nutrition Journal* 10 (9). doi:10.1186/1475-2891-10-9.

Bacon, Linda, and Lucy Aphramor. 2014. *Body Respect: What Conventional Health Books Get Wrong, Leave Out, and Just Plain Fail to Understand about Weight.* Dallas, TX: BenBella Books.

Brown, Harriet. 2015. *Body of Truth: How Science, History, and Culture Drive Our Obsession with Weight— and What We Can Do About It.* Boston, MA: Da Capo Press.

Brunstrom, Jeffrey M., Jeremy F. Burn, Nicola R. Sell, Jane M. Collingwood, Peter J. Rogers, Laura L. Wilkinson, Elanor C. Hinton, Olivia M. Maynard, and Danielle Ferriday. 2012. "Episodic Memory and Appetite Regulation in Humans." *PLoS One* 7 (12). doi:10.1371/journal.pone.0050707.

David, Marc. 1991. *Nourishing Wisdom: A Mind-Body Approach to Nutrition and Well-Being.* New York: Bell Tower.

David, Marc. 2005. *The Slow Down Diet: Eating for Pleasure, Energy, & Weight Loss.* Rochester, VT: Healing Arts Press.

Katie, Byron. 2002. *Loving What Is: Four Questions that can Change Your Life.* New York: Three Rivers Press.

O'Malley, Mary. 2004. *The Gift of our Compulsions: A Revolutionary Approach to Self-Acceptance and Healing.* Novato, CA: New World Library.

Tolle, Eckhart. 1999. *The Power of Now: A Guide to Spiritual Enlightenment.* Novato, CA: New World Library.

Tribole, Evelyn, and Elyse Resch. 2012. *Intuitive Eating.* 3rd ed. New York: St. Martin's Press.

The next step on your journey to food freedom

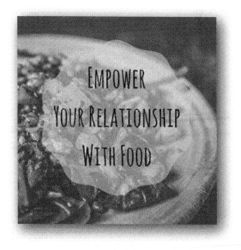

A self-paced course and supportive community that will change your relationship with food—for good!

Visit empower.DawnMacLaughlin.com

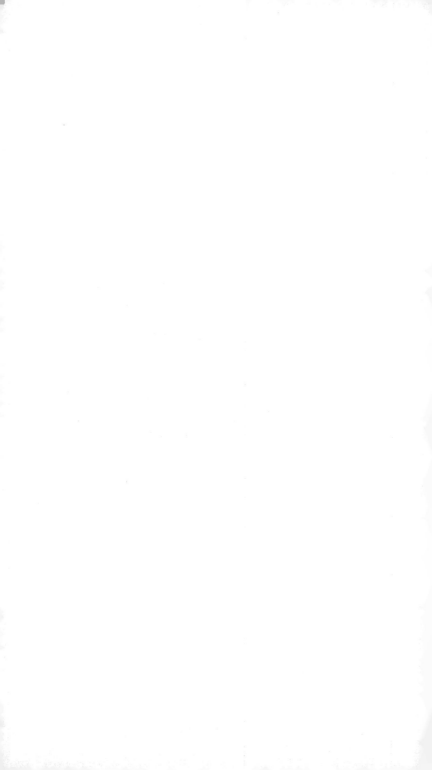

Want to work with me?

I'm on a mission to liberate self-motivated people like you from wasting time, energy, and money on the seemingly perpetual struggle with food, weight, and body so that you feel confident, energized, and alive—without dieting and without giving up the things you love. I offer customized private and group coaching programs to meet you where you are at and get you where you want to go.

Interested? Let's chat. Contact me to schedule a virtual latte at dawn@dawnmaclaughlin.com.

One call could change your life. What are you waiting for?

"Working with Dawn has changed my life completely."
—*Christy*

"Engaging Dawn's services was one of the best decisions I ever made."
—*Jeanie*

"Dawn is much more than a health coach. She is a transformational coach who will help you with every aspect of your life."
—*Renee*

"I am finally free of the mental obsession with food I struggled with all my life."
—*KD*

Want Free Stuff?

To receive weekly tips, recipes, articles, motivational
moments, and other stimulating content,

subscribe to the

Food Freedom Newsletter!

Sign up at FreeGiftFromDawn.com

69521828R00093

Made in the USA
Columbia, SC
16 August 2019